NOURISHED BY DESIGN

NOURISHED BY DESIGN

A Christ-Centered Approach to Nutrition

ANDY FELTON

Printed in the United States of America
First edition, fifth printing. Updated February 2026.

ISBN 979-8-9924713-0-4 (Hardcover)
ISBN 979-8-9924713-1-1 (Softcover)
ISBN 979-8-9924713-2-8 (eBook)

Contents

Author's Disclosures

The author approaches this work from the perspective of the Reformed Protestant Christian tradition, yet every effort has been made to ensure that the content remains relevant and accessible to believers from a wide variety of traditions adhering to historic Christian doctrine. The aim is to present biblically grounded principles that transcend denominational boundaries, encouraging thoughtful engagement and unity among all followers of Christ.

This book is for informational and educational purposes only and is not intended to provide medical advice, diagnose health conditions, or serve as a substitute for professional medical care. Always consider consulting with a qualified healthcare practitioner before making any changes to your diet, supplements, or lifestyle, particularly if you have existing health conditions or are taking medications. The author disclaims any liability for decisions made based on the information provided herein.

Foreword

by Joel Salatin

If you're a Christian, are you embarrassed by mainstream environmentalists who would rather save a tree than an unborn baby? If you're an environmentalist, are you embarrassed by Christians who crusade for the sanctity of life but then buy Happy Meals?

I've lived my whole life in this tension, creating ire among my church friends for being consumed with creation stewardship while facing the disbelief of my organic farming friends that I could claim "the Bible instructs me this way." In numerous media interviews, reporters ask incredulously, "How can you care about the environment *and* be a Christian?"

So wide is the cultural chasm between these two philosophies that the conservative faith community demonizes nearly everything associated with earth care. By and large, American churches embrace genetically modified organisms (GMOs). Church nurseries and Vacation Bible Schools feed snacks of junk food and chemical-laced, Red Dye 29-implanted goodies. Youth groups routinely feast on pizza and Coke. The average churchgoer's home refrigerator is well stocked with squeezable cheese, ultra-processed convenience foods, and sugary soft drinks. But at prayer time, the requests come thick and fast for the conventional maladies that beset the average junk-eating person.

I've been accosted many times by Christians for opposing factory farming, glyphosate, and chemical fertilizer. "It's all going to burn eventually, and we're supposed to dominate," they say with pious platitudes.

I finally wrote a book, *The Marvelous Pigness of Pigs*, to defend a Biblically mandated ethic of creation stewardship. Many Christians have responded positively, saying, "I knew something was wrong, but I didn't have the information to defend myself." The result of all this tension is that creation stewardship gets short shrift in most churches. And if an earth-caring person dares to question the Styrofoam plates at the potluck or the KFC bucket of chicken, the elders quickly step in to silence things. "Are you some sort of creation-worshipping tree hugger, earth muffin, commie pinko?" End of discussion.

My fundamental question is this: Does God care? Does God care about how we raise our chickens? Does God care how we produce corn? If God cares about a sparrow falling and a hair falling out of our head, surely He cares about the life of a pig or a cabbage. And if He cares because it's all His stuff, do you think He has a plan for doing it right or doing it wrong? These are profound thoughts about agriculture and how we treat the earth.

How thrilling to have the next permutation of this theme: does God care about what we eat? In *Nourished by Design*, Andy Felton dares to challenge us to eat Eucharistically. He's taken this theme of earth care from the big picture of creation and farming all the way to the plate, to our food, to our physical bodies.

He ties food directly to our health and dares to ask: is the food I'm eating helping to build soil or depleting it? But more than that, he dives deep into how the body functions, noting that we each carry a health bank account. He suggests that Hot Pockets are a withdrawal, while whole grass-based raw milk is a deposit. This book has a gem on almost every page.

For example, did you know that we have hundreds to thousands of mitochondria per cell, each with a little biological turbine spinning at 96,000 revolutions per minute to create cellular fuel? When I was in high school biology, we looked at cells and knew about some of their innards, but we sure didn't learn about this. Just think about that for a moment and bask in the glorious truth that we're "fearfully and wonderfully made." The more we learn, the more amazing God's creative genius becomes. How about we begin to approach it with humility and wonder, rather than like a swashbuckling conquistador claiming power and ownership?

Andy goes on to explain that there are some 50,000 copper atoms at the center of each mitochondrion. Meditate on that for a moment and your head will explode. Today's fixation on the gut microbiome is bringing people to an awareness of just how amazing the body is. Andy explains that our gut microbes are the first to get information from the outside world. What kind of information is that? Chemicals? Unknown substances?

"Disease is a formidable adversary that we are commanded to resist, but we can only resist this enemy if we are familiar with it," he notes, challenging Christians to change our eating habits in order to present an "object lesson" of redemptive power to the world. What if our churches defied the conventional health statistics by having fewer diabetics, fewer cancers, fewer heart problems? What if health issues did not dominate our prayer vigils?

Andy dives deep into metabolic dysfunction, the anti-meat movement, and theological threads surrounding feasting and fasting. Every Christian—and every non-Christian—should read this book to grasp our responsibilities and privileges regarding personal stewardship of the vessel that houses the Holy Spirit. To be sure, Andy is not in a food cult. I appreciate the grace he offers for those moments when we must be polite—such as at a relative's birthday party where a cake of uncertain origin is served. If we do most things right, our bodies can handle a few assaults.

And isn't that just the way God's grace works? He offers forgiveness when we fail, knowing we'll often fall short. Our bodies reflect that kind of relationship with our decisions, and we can be forever grateful for that. I'm ecstatic that with this book I have both the science and the philosophy to defend a biblical food ethic. Enjoy.

– **Joel Salatin,** renowned American farmer, advocate for sustainable agriculture, and the author of influential works like *Folks, This Ain't Normal* and *The Marvelous Pigness of Pigs*.

Introduction

*"The central question of every human life is
this: where will I go for my sustenance?"*

– Monsignor James Shea

In the beginning, God placed the first humans in a garden teeming
with life and overflowing with abundant food, where Adam and
Eve freely chose their sustenance; their bodies were nourished, their
hearts were at peace, and their minds were attuned to truth. But a
serpent poisoned this banquet. Tempted by a lie, Adam and Eve tasted
the forbidden fruit and from that moment, the appetites of their bodies,
minds, and hearts were distorted.

Humanity, estranged from God, stumbled through an era of
spiritual and physical malnutrition, seeking to satisfy an insatiable
hunger and thirst in ways that only left them emptier. In an attempt to
overcome their alienation, they began offering food sacrifices—sheep,
goats, and the first fruits of their fields—hoping these offerings might
bridge the painful distance between them and God.

But God's favor fell upon Abraham, a man who trusted His plan
and would bear a redemptive promise. In his travels, Abraham met
a mysterious priest named Melchizedek, who offered him bread and
wine—a sacred feast, its full meaning still unknown. In time, Abraham's
grandson, Jacob, secured his famished brother's birthright with a bowl

1

of warm lentil soup. Later named Israel, Jacob would become the father of a nation.

Israel's sons, however, betrayed their brother Joseph, selling him into slavery. Famine drove them back to him, now a ruler in Egypt who had filled its granaries with grain. In a twist of divine providence, Joseph became their savior, feeding the very ones who had abandoned him. What began as refuge in Egypt turned to bondage, and generations later, Moses rose to lead them out of captivity to worship God as a people set apart.

In the wilderness, God gave them water from a rock and bread from the ground, teaching them to depend on Him and to discipline their hunger. Yet the manna, miraculous as it was, soon lost its allure. The people grumbled, yearning for the rich flavors of Egypt. Many perished in discontent, but their descendants entered a promised land—a land overflowing with milk and honey, teeming with wheat and barley, heavy with grapes, figs, and pomegranates. It was a place where all of Israel's needs would be met, so long as they hungered for God above all. When they turned away, seeking satisfaction apart from Him, they fell again into cycles of captivity and despair.

Then, God intervened definitively—not through signs and prophets alone, but by stepping into history as flesh and blood. Born in Bethlehem, the "House of Bread," Jesus was laid in a feeding trough—a striking image of provision for a hungry world. As He grew, He fasted for forty days in the wilderness, emerging physically weak but spiritually unshaken. From this place of hunger, He fed thousands with loaves and fish, turned water into wine, and welcomed everyone to eat and drink freely, as though fasting were a distant concern in His presence.

Jesus told His friends that He had bread they knew nothing about, urging them to pray for it daily. Then, in the fullness of time, He revealed the true food for which they were starving: Himself. One night, He broke bread and shared wine with His friends, calling them His body and blood. The next day, He hung on a tree, crying out in thirst. Few understood that this tree—the cross—was in full bloom, laden with the perfect fruit that would reverse the curse of Eden's forbidden tree and redeem humanity's hunger.

Planted in the ground, this fruit burst forth on the third day, alive and flourishing. The risen Christ was recognized in the breaking of bread on the road to Emmaus and by the shore, where He greeted His disciples with a simple invitation: "Who wants breakfast?"[1]

The Bible, at its core, is a story about food—or more precisely, about hungers satisfied.

God is complete in Himself, but every created thing has needs. This is especially true of humans, the most complex of God's creatures. We have a basic, animalistic need to replenish our physical bodies, but we also yearn to quench our minds' thirst for truth and satisfy our hearts' longings for meaning. In essence, we were designed to depend wholly on God for every aspect of our sustenance—our true "daily bread."

Yet Christians are sometimes tempted by a long-standing misconception: that the Christian life revolves solely around satisfying spiritual hunger, divorced from the physical world.

Under the law, the Israelites were given dietary codes, purification rituals, and sacrificial offerings—a way of life in which worship and obedience shaped every aspect of daily existence. Faith was not merely an internal belief but was embodied in the rhythms of eating, working, resting, and gathering. In contrast, many modern believers tend to treat faith as an abstract or private matter, disconnected from the practical, tangible patterns of daily living.

Ironically, however, when we neglect the physical in favor of the spiritual, it is our spiritual lives that suffer. Few articulated this truth better than American theologian and philosopher Francis Schaeffer, who argued that *true* spirituality is anything but an abstract, disembodied, inner experience. As he puts it:

> "The Christian life, true spirituality, always begins inside but it must be practiced in the external world. The true Christian

---

1   The summary of the Bible story through the lens of food was inspired by and largely adapted from a speech by Monsignor James Shea at the National Eucharistic Conference on July 18, 2024.

life … is not only spiritual but also material. The total person is redeemed, including the physical body, and this body must live out God's truth."[2]

According to Schaeffer, a genuine knowledge of God raises an unavoidable question: "How should we then live?"[3]

If we were to seriously consider this question for all areas of our lives, we would find that, even under the New Covenant, God cares about where we look to satisfy our physical hunger. Sure, this hunger is only a part of our total hunger, but it's no less real or significant. In fact, since true spirituality is a whole person endeavor, how we satisfy our physical hunger plays no small role in shaping and satisfying our other hungers as well. How we secure, prepare, and eat food—central aspects of our embodied existence—reflect how we regard God's created order. These choices reveal whether we truly honor His designs, love His people, and steward His provision—whether we are open to total dependence on our Creator.

Christian farmer and author Joel Salatin argues that attempting to nourish ourselves apart from God's design has led many Christians into a crisis of hypocrisy. He observes that while many Western churchgoers unabashedly affirm God's perfect design when it comes to cultural issues like abortion, marriage, and pornography, we fail to do the same for our diets. Salatin highlights that most Christians act as though they find nothing wrong with participating in worldly food systems that treat God's living creations as mechanical and manipulable and, as we'll explore later, tend to pillage God's created order and disregard His design for human health, relationships, and flourishing.

Salatin pulls no punches, saying, "In our self-righteousness, Christians could make jokes about animal rights, organic farmers,

---

2   Francis A. Schaeffer, *True Spirituality* (Wheaton, IL: Tyndale House Publishers, 1971).

3   This is the title of one of Schaeffer's best-known works.

and fruit and nut eaters, all while holding our Bibles in one hand and gobbling Hot Pockets with the other."[4]

A faith like this—a disembodied, abstract faith—cannot be what God has in mind. We know this because the Gospel reveals a kind spirituality that is no more abstract than Jesus's own life in the flesh. It took the *embodiment* of Truth to redeem mankind. It took God's divine love expressed in time, space, and matter—in human flesh—to show us how we are supposed to live. This revelation reinforces the inescapable conclusion that our eternal, spiritual relationship with God is expressed daily in how we live every aspect of our temporal, physical lives. In Salatin's words, "Our stewardship of things we can see illustrates our stewardship of things we can't see."[5] If we fail to approach our bodies, our food, our health, and God's creation as gifts to be faithfully stewarded according to His design—and worse yet, if we don't see this as a problem—then we are attempting to satisfy our hungers in the wrong way.

It is safe to assume that nutrition is rarely, if ever, explored in most Christian churches. Many believers have probably never heard a sermon or participated in a Bible study on the subject. If they have, it's likely to have been superficial, unsatisfying, or perhaps unbiblical. Yet a large and seemingly growing portion of the Church's prayer requests are for one illness after another, most of them chronic and preventable.

This anecdotal experience mirrors the broader decline in health: More than half of Americans regularly take prescription medications—four, on average[6]—and the adult obesity rate is projected to reach 50 percent in the near future.[7] Despite spending 20 percent of its economic output on health care, America leads the world in deaths from chronic,

---

4   Joel Salatin, *The Marvelous Pigness of Pigs: Respecting and Caring for All God's Creation* (New York: FaithWords, 2016).

5   Ibid.

6   Consumer Reports National Research Center's nationally representative survey of 1,947 adults, conducted in April 2017.

7   Zachary J. Ward, Michael W. Long, Stephen C. Resch, Catherine M. Cradock, and Steven L. Gortmaker. "Projected U.S. State-Level Prevalence of Adult Obesity and Severe Obesity," *New England Journal of Medicine* 381, no. 25 (2019): 2440-2450.

noninfectious diseases and ranks last in the developed world in maternal and infant mortality, behind even most poor African nations.[8] Most alarmingly, our children are increasingly experiencing "adult" diseases, with about 20 percent of adolescents suffering from pre-diabetes.[9] Alongside these outcomes, we see the deterioration of our land, our environment, and our culture, yet we often overlook the connection between these issues and nutrition—an area where Western confusion cries out for the Church's example.

The good news, and the central thesis of this book, is that an applied theology of nutrition centered on Jesus—the Redeemer of the Body, the Bread of Life, and the Divine Physician—can remedy this confusion and offer healing for its many consequences.

Before we explore this applied theology of nutrition, however, we should step back and better understand how we got here.

There's no single "smoking gun" behind our modern nutritional catastrophe. Yet if we doubt the potential societal impact of a theology of nutrition—even a misguided one—we need only look at the remarkable influence of the Seventh-day Adventist (SDA) Church.

Ellen White, a prominent founder of this Protestant denomination, placed healthy living at the center of her denomination's message. Her convictions that "our bodies are Christ's purchased possession" and that "obedience to the laws of health is a matter of personal duty" are, as we'll see, themes that undoubtedly resonate with Christian doctrine.[10] However, her deep conviction that meat eating is detestable to God— that meat is a toxic stimulant that stirs humanity's baser passions and animalistic tendencies—is quite controversial.

---

8   Munira Z. Gunja, Evan D. Gumas, Reginald D. Williams II, "U.S. Health Care from a Global Perspective, 2022: Accelerating Spending, Worsening Outcomes," *Commonwealth Fund*, January 2023, https://www.commonwealthfund.org/publications/issue-briefs/2023/jan/us-health-care-global-perspective-2022.

9   Leah J. Andes, Yiling J. Cheng, David B. Rolka, Edward W. Gregg, and Giuseppina Imperatore. "Prevalence of Prediabetes Among Adolescents and Young Adults in the United States, 2005-2016." *JAMA Pediatrics* 174, no. 2 (2020): e194498.

10   Ellen G. White, *The Ministry of Healing* (Mountain View, CA: Pacific Press Publishing Association, 1905).

White's general view that appetite and taste are unreliable guides for nourishing the body led her to advocate for a plain, simple, vegan diet—a "Garden of Eden" diet—as the ideal. She believed this diet could meet physical needs without inviting the moral corruption that might compromise one's physical and spiritual union with Christ.[11]

While today's nutritional confusion is a far cry from White's simple, wholesome, and temperate advice, it's clear in retrospect that her fingerprints are all over the autopsy of the Western diet.

The ubiquity of breakfast cereals, for example, is due in part to her influence on John Harvey Kellogg, a young Adventist with whom she was so impressed that she sponsored his medical education. White put Kellogg in charge of the Battle Creek Sanitarium, where he researched treatments and developed foods in keeping with Adventist dietary principles.

Kellogg, too, promoted a simple, bland, high-fiber diet for his patients, convinced that meat, which he believed to be the devil incarnate, was the cause of both constipation and masturbation—his chief medical nemeses. While many of his experimental treatments were peculiar, if not downright heinous,[12] his lasting impact lies in the field of nutrition.

Kellogg often experimented with new breakfast cereals and plant-based meat substitutes. For instance, he created oatmeal and cornmeal biscuits that, when broken into pieces, became a popular treat known as "granola." This concoction somewhat controversially inspired one of Kellogg's students, C.W. Post, to start his own cereal empire. Kellogg's big break, however, came when he and his entrepreneurial brother introduced and marketed "Corn Flakes"—the epitome of bland, plant-based, easily digestible food. Of course, both the Kellogg's and Post

---

11   In contrast, the nutritional paradigm presented in this book highlights taste as one of the most appropriate guides to a proper diet. The proper enjoyment of food is among our highest goods, and it both cultivates and reflects our enjoyment of God.

12   Kellogg's treatments included electrocution, fifteen-gallon enemas, vibrating chairs, circumcision without anesthetic, and 46 different types of baths, as he documented in *Plain Facts for the Old and Young*, Middlesex, UK: Echo Library, 1879 (as cited in Robert H. Lustig, *Metabolical: The Lure and the Lies of Processed Food, Nutrition, and Modern Medicine* (New York: Harper Wave, 2021).).

brands would go on to establish and dominate the breakfast cereal industry.

But the SDA Church's nutritional influence goes far beyond the overhaul of traditional breakfast foods. In fact, the denomination was largely responsible for establishing the field of nutrition as an accredited science in the first place.

In 1917, after studying dietetics under Kellogg's mentorship, Adventist Lenna Cooper co-founded the Academy of Nutrition and Dietetics (AND), now the largest organization of nutrition professionals in the United States. Not surprisingly, she embraced her denomination's plant-based, high-carbohydrate diet and contributed greatly to its popularity.[13] But more importantly, the formalization of nutrition and dietetics as technical sciences has profoundly influenced the way we perceive and think about food.

Before these professions were established, *gastronomy* was the leading field related to food and nourishment. Jean Anthelme Brillat-Savarin, a French lawyer and politician in the early nineteenth century, most famously explored the art and science of gastronomy in his best-known work, *The Physiology of Taste*. He described the field as "the reasoned comprehension of everything connected with the nourishment of man," driven by an appreciation for the proper enjoyment of food—the flavors, textures, and quality of ingredients, as well as the cultural and traditional aspects that food highlights and refines.[14]

Brillat-Savarin didn't know what calories were. In fact, no one really knew what calories were until nutrition moved away from the study of flavor and culture and to the science of metabolism.

One of the pioneers of this shift was Wilbur Atwater, an American chemist known for his work in calorimetry. Atwater was the first to calculate the caloric energy content of the three main macronutrients—carbohydrates, fats, and proteins (4, 9, and 4 calories per gram,

---

13 Cooper famously coined the phrase, "breakfast is the most important meal of the day" in *Good Health* magazine, a publication edited by Kellogg himself.

14 Jean Anthelme Brillat-Savarin, *The Physiology of Taste: Or, Meditations on Transcendental Gastronomy*, trans. M. F. K. Fisher (New York: Counterpoint, 1999).

respectively)—by measuring the chemical energy they release when incinerated. Dietitians, recognizing the practical appeal of this approach, coined the "calories in, calories out" method, which tends to demonize fat (the most calorically dense macronutrient) and reduces nutrition to a simple math equation, overlooking the complexities of digestion and how the body uses food.

By the 1970's, nutrition science had evolved beyond basic calorie counting and was applying research to emerging diseases and health issues. Much of this research had coalesced around the idea that saturated fat, cholesterol, and sodium were the primary contributors to heart disease. Given the association of these nutrients with fatty animal products, especially meat, this perspective fit well with the SDA Church's dietary views and gained support through its influence in the fields of nutrition and dietetics. Loma Linda University, the research arm of the Adventist Church, significantly contributed to the popularity of the theory with a series of influential studies.[15]

In 1977, the US government enshrined this theory into law with the initial publication of the Dietary Guidelines. These guidelines, which have remained largely unchanged since, stigmatized dietary fat (especially saturated fat), called for a 50–85 percent reduction in salt intake, recommended a daily limit of 300 milligrams of dietary cholesterol, and, most notably, encouraged people to make carbohydrates 55–60 percent of their daily caloric intake.[16]

It is perhaps no coincidence that Nick Mottern, the congressional aide widely credited with drafting these guidelines, was both a devout Adventist and a vegetarian who relied upon Loma Linda University's research as evidence for his claims.

These precise, supposedly research-backed recommendations stand in contrast to Brillat-Savarin's more wholesome advice, encapsulated in

---

15   The Adventist Health Study of 1958, for example, provided an in-depth look at the health outcomes of Adventists, many whom followed vegetarian diets. This research provided evidence supporting the benefits of plant-based diets in reducing the risk of heart disease.

16   United States Senate Select Committee on Nutrition and Human Needs, *Dietary Goals for the United States,* (US Government Printing Office, 1977).

such whimsical quotes as, "A dessert without cheese is like a beautiful woman with only one eye." But he, jokes aside, had a far better understanding of nutrition than Washington bureaucrats.

Even the most "primitive" cultures have historically demonstrated a far deeper, more practical understanding of nutrition than our modern orthodoxy. In the early twentieth century, Cleveland dentist Weston A. Price traveled the globe studying traditional peoples whom the modern world might have dismissed as backward. From Swiss villagers in remote valleys to African tribes in the highlands, these cultures had little in common—except for two remarkable features: magnificent health marked by strong teeth and well-formed bone structures, and diets entirely free of industrialized foods. Their regional staples differed widely, but all shared a near-sacred reverence for nutrient-dense food. They observed strict dietary practices for fertility and childbearing and clearly understood the consequences of straying from the wisdom handed down through the generations.

Price published his famous findings in 1939, yet our nutritional establishment continues its march in the opposite direction, now armed with ever more sophisticated tools, like the *Food Compass*, developed from a 2021 study by Tufts University. This advanced nutritional profiling system compiles data on disease risk factors and assigns foods a healthiness score from 1 to 100 based on their nutrient content, processing methods, and other attributes. According to this system, "eggs cooked in butter" score a measly 29, flagged for minimization in the diet. However, a bowl of Kellogg's Raisin Bran (72), drenched in skim milk (18 points higher than whole milk) and accompanied by a glass of apple juice (55) is considered a much healthier choice. The contrast couldn't be more stark. As this book will soon show, highly processed sugar flakes covered in skimmed, ultra-pasteurized, and homogenized milk with a glass of diabetes juice on the side is a metabolic cluster bomb—far from God's design for our nourishment. Buttery eggs, on the other hand, may as well be the gold standard.

Markets and social trends have eagerly aligned with government-sanctioned nutritional advice promoted by the Food Compass—advice that has proven highly profitable for Big Food. The demonization of traditional cooking fats like butter and lard, for instance, paved the way for ultra-processed alternatives like soybean, canola, and sunflower oils, once considered industrial waste or used as machine lubricants. Stripped of any trace of their living origins, these oils are ideal for creating long-lasting, shelf-stable products. But despite their toxic effects in the body, which we'll outline later, they have largely escaped the scrutiny of any influential institutions.[17]

Similarly, the removal of natural fats from many foods made large amounts of refined sugar a near necessity to compensate for lost flavor. The consumption of refined sugars and grains, a rare luxury in past societies, is now perhaps the most common addiction in the West.

These trends largely coincided with the "Green Revolution" of the 1940s–60s, a period of agricultural transformation that upended small, diverse family farms and rural farming communities out of a perceived need for industrialization to feed the world's growing population. This movement, though seemingly well-intentioned, justified the abandonment of time-honored agricultural practices—like crop rotation, natural fertilization, and human and animal labor—in favor of herbicides, fossil-fuel-based fertilizers, genetically modified crops, and industrial machinery. With subsidies from the US Farm Bill, Big Food has transformed the historically unprofitable monoculture of corn, soy, and wheat into a powerhouse for the processed food industry, poisoning the soil, the food, and the people who eat it.

While each of these developments has contributed to our overall decline in health—a topic we'll discuss in depth—this book is no exposé; much of this information is already widely known. So why, after half a century, have these missteps gone largely unaddressed? Why does the government continue to support biologically poisoned commodity crops

---

17   The American Heart Association, for example, continues to promote canola, soybean, corn, and sunflower seed oils (American Heart Association, "Dietary Fats," last modified January 18, 2023, https://www.heart.org/en/healthy-living/healthy-eating/eat-smart/fats/dietary-fats.).

that are turned into all kinds of ultra-processed foods and distributed in school lunches and food assistance programs?

As with many other perpetually broken systems, a key factor is the distorted incentive structure driven by powerful financial interests.

Calley Means, a former Big Food strategy consultant, provides a relevant and unfortunate example of the ultra-processed food industry's playbook with this revealing testimony:

> "Early in my career, I consulted for Coke to fight back against sugar taxes in Pennsylvania. We first identified the most influential African American pastors in the state. Coke then (confidentially) donated millions of dollars to them. The pastors then held press conferences, saying sugar taxes were racist. The media covered it, racial tensions flared, and Coke defeated the taxes."[18]

With that kind of influence, it's no coincidence that 10 percent of the food dollars for families on taxpayer-funded food stamps are spent on sugary drinks.[19] Is it any wonder that, presumably for the first time in world history, those with the lowest incomes have the highest rates of obesity?[20]

Furthermore, the Academy of Nutrition and Dietetics is funded by junk food companies, holds stock in ultra-processed food giants, and has a well-documented history of quid pro quo arrangements with the industry.[21] Even nutrition research is not immune to this influence:

18   Calley Means, "Free Market?" December 29, 2022, https://calleymeans.com/2022/12/29/free-market/.

19   Allison Aubrey, "Food Stamps for Soda: Time to End Billion-Dollar Subsidy for Sugary Drinks," *NPR*, October 29, 2018, https://www.npr.org/sections/thesalt/2018/10/29/659634119/food-stamps-for-soda-time-to-end-billion-dollar-subsidy-for-sugary-drinks.

20   Cynthia L. Ogden, Tala H. Fakhouri, Margaret D. Carroll, et al., "Prevalence of Obesity Among Adults, by Household Income and Education — United States, 2011–2014," *MMWR Morbidity and Mortality Weekly Report* 66 (2017): 1369–1373.

21   Tom Perkins, "Revealed: Group Shaping US Nutrition Receives Millions From Big Food Industry," *The Guardian*, December 9, 2022, https://www.theguardian.com/science/2022/dec/09/academy-nutrition-financial-ties-processed-food-companies-contributions?s=09.

the Food Compass study was directly funded by the food conglomerate Danone and indirectly supported by the Food and Nutrition Innovation Council, a coalition that includes major players like PepsiCo, Kraft Heinz, and Nestlé.

Casey and Calley Means, in their book *Good Energy*, argue that every institution that affects health—from Big Food to Big Pharma, from hospitals to medical schools, and even insurance companies—profits more from society's perpetual sickness than from its health.

In sum, perhaps our poor health outcomes result from an alliance of flawed policy, misguided science, and perverse financial interests, all influenced at least in part by questionable religious dogma.

Renowned physician and author Robert Lustig argues that the solution to this conundrum is to remove religion from the equation, lamenting that "the science of nutrition has been co-opted by the religion of nutrition." If we could strip away the dogma, he suggests, and examine the science objectively, we might find that various dietary approaches, ranging from vegan to keto, are all viable options.[22]

To Lustig's credit, he may be on to something—but he also misses the core issue. The problem is not simply the intrusion of religious dogma into nutrition but the mistaken belief that science can function as both the target and the means of getting there—that it can tell us not only how to proceed but where we ought to go. Science can measure and describe, but it cannot answer the most fundamental questions: What is health for? What is the body for? What are we for?

These are questions of meaning, purpose, and value—questions that science is not equipped to answer because they lie outside its scope. They are not scientific questions; they are philosophical and theological questions.

As Leon Kass, physician, scientist, and philosopher, insightfully observes:

---

22   Robert Lustig, *Metabolical*, (Harper, 2021), pg. 75-76.

"We are today, before the large human questions, like men lost at sea without a compass. We adhere to a science that provides us with enormous power to travel but that denies the existence of knowledge about who we are and where we should go."[23]

Nutrition—a reflection on the body, food, and health—is inseparable from these larger questions about human life and purpose. As Kass points out, it is a mistake to imagine that nutrition can be rightly understood apart from a worldview.

The solution, then, is not to pretend we have no presuppositions, but to recognize that we do—and to ensure that they are the *right* ones. In other words, if we point our "food compass" directly at Jesus—the perfect revelation of nutrition—and use science as one of many tools to propel us, we may actually be on to something.

This book is neither a forty-day health devotional nor a biblical weight-loss plan, nor does it assume that God's design for nutrition is found in any one historical diet from the Bible. Rather, in the following chapters, we'll seek to build a meaningful paradigm for nutrition—not because the Bible offers a comprehensive manual on diet or health, but precisely because it does not. While many passages have been misused to promote modern Western ideals of fitness and diet, the Bible actually speaks sparingly and indirectly about what to eat or how to pursue health. For most of church history, such questions rarely demanded theological reflection. But in an age of industrialized food, chronic disease, and profound confusion about the body, we are left with a gap that must be addressed. To do so faithfully, we must draw from the whole counsel of Scripture, as well as from science and tradition, to recover a framework that honors God's design.

We'll begin by considering the proper meaning of the body, food, and health to establish the worldview from which to approach the scientific research. We'll then dive into a practical understanding of our metabolic health, how it goes awry, and how we can support it with

---

23   Leon R. Kass, *The Hungry Soul: Eating and the Perfecting of Our Nature,* (Chicago: University of Chicago Press, 1999), Pg. 8.

the foods God designed for our nourishment. Finally, we'll refine this understanding, further connecting it to some of the larger questions that animate the Christian life: How should we think about feasting and fasting? What does the Bible actually say about eating meat? And what are the broader implications of the food systems in which we participate?

This book is an invitation to humbly, cautiously, and yet optimistically transform the mundane act of eating into a means not only of regaining more energy, strength, and vitality, but also of developing and satisfying a hunger for more than food—for God himself.

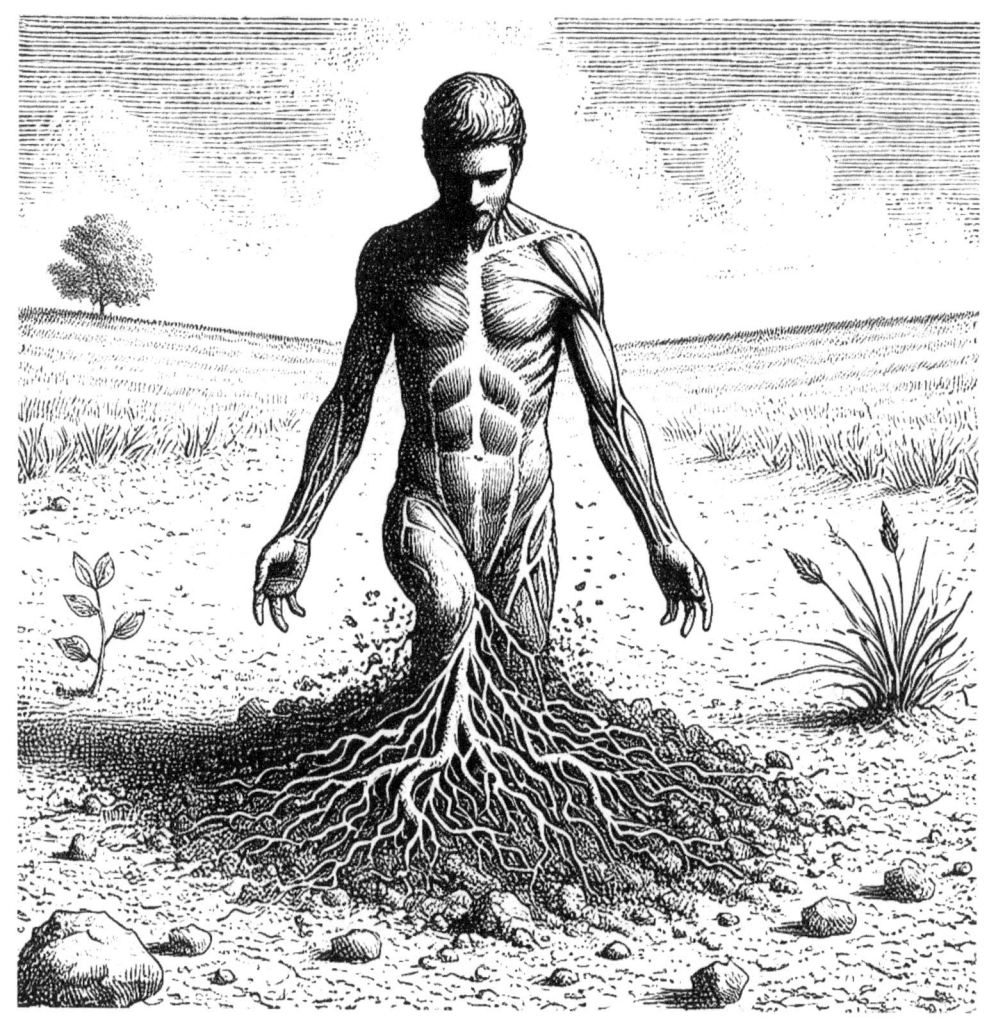

PART I

A Theology of Nutrition

"God never meant man to be a purely spiritual creature. That is why he uses material things like bread and wine to put the new life into us. We may think this rather crude and unspiritual. God does not: He invented eating. He likes matter. He invented it."

– C.S. Lewis, *Mere Christianity*

T hinking about nutrition inevitably brings to mind the time-worn adage "You are what you eat." This phrase has so thoroughly infiltrated our collective consciousness that it has almost become a cliché. Few people, however, are aware of its origins. It was Jean Anthelme Brillat-Savarin, the famous gastronome, who coined the original version: "Tell me what you eat, and I shall tell you what you are."[24]

The intuitive appeal of the concept has led to its resonance across diverse worldviews. Most notably, the atheist German philosopher Ludwig Feuerbach adapted it into "Man is what he eats," a variant that is closer to the modern English rendition.[25] Feuerbach used this expression to encapsulate his materialistic philosophy: humans are as material as the food they eat, and nothing more.

This interpretation contrasts sharply with Brillat-Savarin's original conception, which was consistent with his view of food as a divine gift to be savored. In his eyes, to be a "gourmand" was a prestigious distinction. It signified a person who had transcended the role of a mere eater to become a connoisseur—someone who found deep, almost spiritual meaning in the sensory delights of a meticulously prepared meal. He astutely noted that some devout Christians were among the finest foodies, suggesting a link between spiritual devotion and an appreciation for the transcendental aspects of dining.

The phrase gained widespread popularity in the English language during the 1940s, thanks to American nutritionist Victor Lindlahr. His book, *You Are What You Eat: How to Win and Keep Health with Diet*, cemented the saying as a succinct expression of the relationship between diet and health.

However, the phrase's playful tone can sometimes obscure its profound implications. At first glance, "You are what you eat" seems to comment only on the body's metabolic process: the body converts food into nutrients, which are then reassembled into the body's shape. But a deeper look reveals more complex questions: Are our dietary choices

---

24   Brillat-Savarin, *The Physiology of Taste.*
25   Ludwig Feuerbach, *Concerning Spiritualism and Materialism* (1863).

integral to our identity? Does altering our diet change who we are? What is the relationship between the physical body and the person as a whole? How do we distinguish between the body's ever-changing material and its constant form? And how do the mind, soul, and spirit interact within this framework, assuming they exist at all?

This rabbit hole is enough to make one's head spin, but these questions and their implications become intelligible when understood according to a comprehensive worldview. Therefore, the following four chapters are devoted to laying the foundation for nutrition according to the Christian worldview.

In laying this theological groundwork, it becomes evident that Scripture does not provide a concise manual for nutrition. It does, however, consistently bear witness to the fundamental principles upon which a theology of nutrition can be constructed.

According to the Cambridge dictionary, nutrition is defined as "the substances that you take into your *body* as *food* and the way that they influence your *health*."[26] Within this definition, three interrelated components—the body, food, and health—each have profound theological significance and thus serve as the focal points of this paradigm.

We must first come to grips with the human body, uncovering its meaning, purpose, and relationship to personhood. Scripture repeatedly emphasizes the holistic nature of humanity—comprising mind, body, and soul. This underscores the imperative that no field of study, nutrition included, should treat the body or its members in isolation from the whole person. By meditating further on what constitutes the body in the first place, we are left with a framework from which to understand the importance of food.

The subsequent exploration of food underscores the notion that God is fundamentally concerned with our nourishment. Our inherent dependence as creatures compels us to rely upon God as the source of

---

26   *Cambridge Dictionary*, s.v. "nutrition," accessed September 4, 2024, https://dictionary. cambridge.org.

all sustenance, graciously provided in abundance as a reflection of His self-offering love. Just as the body is made of food, Scripture stresses that individuals are built and continually rebuilt through both material and spiritual nourishment. The Old Testament lays the foundation for these realities, which ultimately find their fulfillment in Christ, whose flesh is called "true food" and whose blood is called "true drink" (Jn. 6:55). By viewing the Lord's Supper as the epitome of human nourishment, we uncover perspectives that can be applied to eating in a broader context.

Lastly, by applying the foundational understanding of humanity's integrated nature and the significance of nourishment, we can delve into a theology of health. A precise definition of health allows us to integrate the concept into a broader framework of Christian living.

It is important to note that this theology does not adopt a "health and wealth" perspective, since health should not be perceived as an end in itself or an earthly reward for a strong faith. Properly understood, however, health is very much like a form of wealth; it can and should be seen as a resource, just like our finances. By acknowledging the eternal implications of our stewardship of God's resources, we can properly understand the moral significance of our duty to steward our health and conclude that an investment in a healthy body is a facilitator of other virtuous Christian pursuits that pay dividends for our *eternal* wealth.

In short, this section will argue that while "you are what you eat" captures part of the truth, a distinctly Christian framework for nutrition recognizes that our identities in Christ hinge much more on *who* we eat, *how* we eat, and *what we do* with the strength we receive from our diets.

1

Nourishing the Temple
(A Theology of the Body)

*"To live is to be in a body in a place joined to
all the bodies of creation. It is our life but it is
also the life God chose for himself in the body of
Jesus. Embodiment is not alien to God, nor is it a
reality only temporarily (and thus begrudgingly)
assumed. Bodies are the places and the means
of God's creating and sustaining love."*

– NORMAN WIRZBA, *FOOD AND FAITH*

The field of nutrition has long focused on the inner workings of metabolism, studying the physical and chemical interactions between our organs and the food we eat. We analyze the role of certain hormones in liver function, investigate how enzymes break down carbohydrates in the digestive tract, and study the absorption and utilization of vitamins and minerals by our cells. In short, nutrition typically focuses on *how* the metabolism works.

Occasionally, it goes beyond the how to explore the *why* behind certain metabolic processes. Rarely, however, does it consider the *who*—the person, the organic whole that is the true subject of these chemical interactions and the organizing principle toward which they are directed. If we seek a nutritional paradigm that honors God and His design, then it is this whole—the human person—that must be the starting point of our inquiry.

In other words, we must ask, "Who is the self that eats?"

What is a Person?

What we seek is a proper anthropology, a task that requires us to first understand our own embodiment and the intricate relationship between body and personhood. While pointy-headed philosophers have long pondered this question, we tend to simply live life without much reflection on the mysteries of our own physical existence, feeling little need to question the essence of our being or the location of our "true selves." This is probably a good thing. But even without realizing it, we engage with some of the most profound metaphysical questions about the body through the language we use every day.

For instance, we often refer to our bodies as if they were separate entities from ourselves. We might say, "My body needs rest," as if a body were simply a vessel. We talk about "listening to the body" or "taking care of our bodies" in ways that subtly imply a divide between the physical and the personal. It's hard to avoid this kind of division in self-referential speech, where the speaker is both the subject and the object, the observer and the observed.[27]

These phrases also imply that the body is a form of property. But how does owning a body compare to, say, owning a car? And if the body is indeed a kind of property, who really owns it?

These questions have become more relevant as modern movements have made phrases like "I am a woman trapped in a man's body" socially acceptable. Who, exactly, is the "I" in this case, and how did this "I" get trapped in the wrong body? If the "I" is merely a collection of thoughts and feelings, then where would we locate

---

27   Leon R. Kass, "Thinking About the Body," *The Hastings Center Report* 15, no. 1 (1985): 20–30.

this individual, and, even more challenging, how would we go about "rescuing" him from this material prison?

Perhaps our everyday use of language raises more questions than it is prepared to resolve. Yet, these questions aren't sufficiently answered even in disciplines like modern philosophy and science.

Many philosophers, especially in psychology and related fields, tend to equate personhood with pure will and reason, as if the body were incidental. This notion has deep roots in dualism, which posits a separation between the material and spiritual realms. Dualists argue that the mind or soul is the metaphysical essence that defines a person's identity, and in some religious beliefs this entity can float away from the material world to eternal life.

In contrast, scientific naturalism—the dominant perspective within the scientific community—requires a materialistic worldview, asserting that all aspects of existence are bound to the physical world. According to materialism, our bodies, thoughts, and actions are the results of purely physical processes that operate only through the deterministic laws of nature. In this view, selfhood is entirely physical and rooted in the body. However, materialism doesn't elevate the body to the dignity of the person; rather, it lowers the person to the dignity of the body, which it sees as nothing more than a lump of matter without animating force or transcendent meaning. While dualists regard will and reason as central to personhood, materialists regard the appearance of free will and reason as an illusion, merely the result of physical and chemical reactions between molecules, devoid of any spiritual component.

In short, both dualism and materialism reduce the human body to a mere sack of meat. For the dualist, this meat sack is the dwelling place of the self, or its clothing. This clothing, if anything, corrupts the transcendent self. For the materialist, the meat sack *is* the self. However, this meat sack is only one of many meat sacks that arise naturally from random and undirected processes. Consequently, materialists regard the body as neither morally reprehensible nor wrong, but rather insignificant and meaningless.

In contrast, Scripture offers a richer and more coherent anthropology. Through a proper theology of the body, we can explore the meaning, purpose, and dignity of the human body within God's design for creation and redemption—an essential foundation for understanding nutrition. As theologian Norman Wirzba beautifully puts it, creation is "the concrete expression of God's hospitable love making room for what is not God to be and to flourish."[28] Within this created order, human beings stand foremost, made in the image and likeness of God—not merely as souls inhabiting bodies, nor as bodies without souls, but as unified composites of both. To grasp this fully, we must return to the beginning, to the opening chapters of Genesis. There, we encounter Adam in his "original solitude," followed by the creation of Eve and a period of "original unity," and finally the distortion—but not the complete dissolution—of this unity through the introduction of original sin.

Original Solitude: The Body Manifests the Person

Genesis presents the creation story in two complementary accounts. The first chapter offers a cosmic view, recalling the creation of humanity as male and female on the sixth day, created in the image of God and given the mandate to "be fruitful and multiply and fill the earth and subdue it" (Gen. 1:28). The second account of creation, told in the second chapter of Genesis, zooms in to focus more intimately on humanity's special role in creation. In stark contrast to the grand and cosmic account, Genesis 2 presents a close-up view of human origins, specifically describing the embodied experience of the first two created humans. Here we encounter, as Pope John Paul II puts it, "the oldest description and record of man's self-understanding and... the first witness of human conscience."[29]

---

28 Norman Wirzba, *Food and Faith: A Theology of Eating*, 2nd ed. (Cambridge: Cambridge University Press, 2019).

29 John Paul II, *Man and Woman He Created Them: A Theology of the Body*, trans. Michael Waldstein (Boston: Pauline Books & Media, 2006), Section 3.1.

In this focused retelling of creation, we first encounter Adam in his "original solitude" as the only rational being on earth. He is "formed... of dust from the ground," sharing a common origin with the animals—a body made of the same stuff. This body allows him to interact with the visible world, but it also sets him apart from it (Gen. 2:7).

As Adam searches for a companion like himself—a search for identity—he finds instead a series of contrasts, becoming increasingly aware of what he is *not*. His first task of naming each creature further underscores this distinction: He is a body among bodies, yet he alone is self-aware and superior to the animals. In naming them, he recognizes that none of them is a suitable companion.

In addition to helping Adam distinguish himself from other creatures and recognize his need for a partner, his body reveals other aspects of his humanity. Specifically, the unique capabilities of the human body provide a picture of what a person *is* by revealing what a person *does*.

This is most clearly seen in man's duty to cultivate and subdue the earth. Before Adam's creation, the land was barren because "there was no man to work the ground" (Gen. 2:5). Only after God forms Adam from dust does He plant and place him in the Garden of Eden, suggesting that Adam's unique authority over the visible world is tied to his ability to cultivate it.

In other words, the design of the human body enables a person to be the "author of genuinely human activity."[30] By analyzing the structure and function of the body, we gain valuable insight into human nature as a whole.

For example, the philosopher Erwin Straus observed decades ago that our upright posture offers insight into humanity's unique interactions with the world.

At first, his observations were largely symbolic: the upright posture reflects humanity's moral capacity and consciousness. This is reflected in language, where "uprightness" is synonymous with moral character—qualities such as honesty, fairness, and righteousness. Upright posture

---

30   Ibid., Section 7:1.

also symbolizes mankind's resistance to nature. Physically, we resist gravity, but symbolically, we resist forces beneath human dignity.

Anatomically, the upright posture relieves our upper limbs of the task of supporting the body, freeing the arms and hands for new tasks. Hands become tools and sensory instruments, serving as the primary interface for human experience. This freedom allows us to perform crafts and activities that are unique to our species and to explore a new spatial dimension—the lateral dimension. Unlike most animals, humans interact with the world in a lateral space, like an imaginary cylinder whose radius extends to the reach of our arms—a neutral zone that serves as an "action space" between ourselves and our surroundings.

The upright posture also raises our eyes and ears off the ground, making vision the dominant sense over smell and hearing. In most animals, the eyes are aligned with the jaws, making the bite a primary interaction with the world, essential for hunting, carrying, and defending. In humans, however, the mouth is placed below the eyes, which look laterally toward the horizon, capable of perceiving, comprehending, and even wondering about what lies near and far. For humans, sight becomes insight, which is capable of being spoken, heard, and understood in all its nuances.[31]

Straus's reflection on the upright posture is deeply philosophical, indeed, but not without practical significance. It is an insightful testament to lived human experience, commenting on the many ways in which the body expresses realities about the person that are more than just physical. In this way, the body has a kind of sacramental dimension, acting as a visible sign of invisible realities and forcing us to resist the idea that it is nothing more than a vessel or an "earth suit" for the person inside.

---

31   Erwin W. Straus, "The Upright Posture," *The Psychiatric Quarterly* 26, no. 1–4 (January 1952): 529–61.

Original Unity: The Body Reveals the Person's Communal Nature

While Adam's original solitude reveals important truths about human nature, it leaves us with only a partial anthropology.

Genesis underscores that humans are unfit to be alone—that Adam cannot fully understand his identity without a suitable helper.[32] This highlights the inherently relational nature of humanity and foreshadows the creation of a partner to fulfill this fundamental human need.

The rest of the story shows that God brings Adam into a state of non-being, from which emerges a "definitive creation"—humanity in its double unity as male and female. Adam immediately recognizes the woman as a body of the same kind, a helper truly fit for him, and the fulfillment of his identity. In awe, he proclaims, "This at last is bone of my bones and flesh of my flesh; she shall be called Woman, because she was taken out of Man." The Scripture goes on to say, "Therefore a man shall leave his father and his mother and hold fast to his wife, and they shall become one flesh" (Gen. 2:23–24).

Adam instinctively understands that she is for him and he is for her—that his humanity is fulfilled through their union.

By creating Eve from Adam's rib rather than from his head or foot, God establishes a relationship of mutual attraction and equality, in which neither seeks to dominate the other.[33] Within this unity, however, a profound duality remains: their masculinity and femininity complement each other, resolving Adam's solitude and yet affirming all that can be known about the human person in that original state.

The unity and communion of persons, most fully realized when man and woman become "one flesh," adds a new dimension to the creation of humanity in the image and likeness of God. The mystery of the Trinity involves one God in three persons—Father, Son, and Holy Spirit—each fully God and yet distinct in personhood. Human nature is most fully expressed through an analogous communion. Humanity

---

32   Genesis 2:18-20.

33   John W. Kleinig, *Wonderfully Made: A Protestant Theology of the Body,* (Bellingham, WA: Lexham Press, 2021), 34.

reflects the image of God not so much in solitude as in communion. From the beginning, man is not simply an image reflecting the solitary dominion of one person, but rather, and more profoundly, the image of an unfathomable divine communion of persons.[34]

Masculinity and femininity reveal the complementary design of the human body, uncovering a purpose that was hidden in Adam's original solitude. The mutually enriching nature of these two counterparts serves as an object lesson in God's own self-giving love, illustrating that human nature is most fully expressed in the total gift of self, beautifully complemented by the willingness to receive the self-gift of another.

Original Nakedness and Shame: The Estranged Body

Finally, much can be learned about God's intent for the human body by contrasting His original design with the consequences of the Fall.

In their original unity, "the man and his wife were both naked and were not ashamed" (Gen. 2:25). This seemingly small detail concludes the Creation account in Genesis 2, but it takes on greater significance after the fall in the next chapter, when temptation leads them to eat the forbidden fruit. Immediately upon doing so, "the eyes of both were opened, and they knew that they were naked" (Gen. 3:7). Thus, the boundary experience of original sin is followed by a profound shift in how they perceive their bodies.

Some suggest that Adam and Eve were simply unaware of their nakedness before the Fall, and that the transition to knowledge marks a departure from blissful ignorance. But this interpretation overlooks the anthropological significance of the text. They were not unaware, like small children, but fully conscious of their original state, delighting in their nakedness, with no need to hide from one another.

Their "naked and unashamed" state reflects instead what Protestant author John Kleinig describes as having "transparent bodies," in which their physical forms perfectly disclosed their inner purity without

---

34   John Paul II, *Man and Woman He Created Them.*

distortion or misrepresentation.[35] Because their minds and souls were unblemished, and because their bodies reflected that purity, they felt no fear of being fully seen. John Paul II describes this state not as a lack of consciousness, but as a "fullness of conscience." Through their bodies, Adam and Eve could physically perceive the meaning of themselves and each other, fully understanding their humanity and personhood, created in God's image.

It is fitting for a book on nutrition that the fall from innocence centers on eating a piece of fruit. While it's tempting to interpret this solely as a lapse in bodily discipline—a corruption of the appetite—this is only part of the story. Eve is tempted to sin with her whole person, experiencing a threefold distortion: her bodily desire for enjoyable food, her mind's craving for greater knowledge, and her soul's wavering trust in God's will.[36]

With the introduction of sin, the originally integrated harmony of the human person is fractured. The body no longer fully reveals the person as it once did; instead, the experience of shame reflects the fear of being objectified, of being seen as something to be used rather than as a person to be loved. The desire to cover the body after the fall— initially with makeshift loincloths of fig leaves—stems directly from this disintegration. The body now struggles to convey the fullness of the self, and vulnerability is coupled with the fear of being misunderstood or exploited. The instinctive way of receiving and participating in the goodness of creation as a gift, of seeing the fruits of life as a sign of their Creator, and of seeing one another clearly, is clouded by the desire to possess and define life on one's own terms.

But while sin distorts the unity of mind, body, and spirit, it doesn't erase their original purpose or the truth that each aspect remains essential to human identity. The body is not a separate entity from the soul or the mind, but remains a vessel for the expression of the person's inner self, however imperfectly it may now do so. This fragmentation therefore calls not for a reassessment of our identity, but for its redemption.

---

35 Kleinig, *Wonderfully Made*, 35.
36 Ibid., 40.

A proper theology of the body challenges the low view of the body offered by advocates of both materialism and dualism. Adam's original solitude reveals profound insights into the nature of the human person; the body serves as the manifestation of the person in time and space, revealing both physical and spiritual aspects of human nature. The creation of mankind's original unity with a complementary design for male and female further reveals the relational dimension of human nature, providing a physical representation of God's spiritual communion of persons. Finally, the experience of the Fall reinforces the idea that God designed us as a harmonious composite of body and soul, a union that sin distorts but cannot completely dissolve.

Why else would the Father have sent His Son in an incarnate, embodied form—and raised Him with an eternal, perfected resurrection body—if not to redeem the whole person, body and soul? In Christ, humanity is invited to repent, be restored, and walk in the freedom of being rightly ordered—where body and soul are brought into greater harmony. But while believers await the full integration of resurrected bodies in the age to come, even now, in these fallen but purposeful bodies, there is dignity and meaning. The body remains central to vocation, communion, and worship—and even in its frailty, it is the instrument through which nourishment, stewardship, and participation in God's good creation take place.

What is a Body?

Having established that the person who eats is an integrated whole of body, mind, and spirit, we must now consider a seemingly simple yet complex question: what exactly *is* a body? This inquiry, far from trivial, has profound implications for how we approach nutrition.

To appreciate the nuances of defining the human body, we must recognize that it's not simply a single organism, but an ecosystem teeming with life. Within and on our skin reside trillions of other beings—the microbiome, a vast collection of microorganisms that live in symbiosis with us. The human body, like other animals, is more accurately described as a "holobiont," consisting of a host inhabited by a diverse array of organisms. However, even this definition isn't entirely accurate, as it implies that a "host" can exist independently. In reality, the relationship between the "host" and its many inhabitants is so intertwined that it's impossible to consider one without the other; our bodies rely on these organisms—throughout the gut, skin, mouth, and respiratory tract—for essential functions in metabolism and immunity. In fact, "non-human" cells outnumber "human" cells in the body, with approximately 1.3 bacterial cells for every human cell, not counting the numerous viruses, fungi, and other organisms we harbor.[37]

The symbiotic role of these microbes is most evident in the gut, where trillions of them break down indigestible fibers, produce short-chain fatty acids and essential nutrients, and help train the immune system. They also release hormones and neurotransmitters that influence metabolism, regulate inflammation, and communicate with the brain—primarily via the vagus nerve—to affect mood, stress response, and overall brain function. This vast community of inhabitants exists because we feed it, and we would do well to be gracious hosts, as these microbes return the favor in countless ways. Yet their populations are in constant flux, with different species multiplying or dying off in a dynamic process that is both competitive and cooperative—forming a rich ecosystem that continually both supports and shapes us from within.

Like our inhabitants, our "stuff" is constantly changing. The elementary particles that make up our bodies are constantly being exchanged, calling into question where one person ends and the rest of creation begins. For example, with each breath, we exchange oxygen for carbon dioxide. Water, which makes up most of our bodies, is constantly lost through sweat, respiration, and urine and must be replenished by drinking. Even our cells, though they last longer than water, are

---

37   Ron Sender et al., "Revised Estimates for the Number of Human and Bacteria Cells in the Body," PLoS Biology 14, no. 8 (August 19, 2016): e1002533.

constantly regenerating as old cells are shed and replaced by new ones built from the nutrients we consume.

The early Greek thinker Empedocles proposed that "of all mortal things there is no birth nor any end in baneful death, but only a mixing and a separation of things mixed," suggesting that nothing exists as a complete whole, but rather as complex systems in a state of perpetual reorganization.[38] This principle finds resonance in a variety of philosophies that, for better or worse, continue to inform the ethos of natural science in the modern age.

Taoism, for example, promotes the concept that all things, including the human body, are in a state of constant flux, emphasizing a natural flow of life. In this view, the body is a microcosm of the universe, mirroring its rhythms of perpetual change. That's why Casey Means, a prominent doctor and author, suggests that the body is not really an *entity*, but rather a *process* in constant renewal. Similarly, biblical imagery that compares man to a fleeting breath echoes this notion, suggesting that we are a transient part of a universe that is constantly in motion and transformation.[39]

The synthesis of these philosophical concepts with contemporary scientific insights invites us to question whether the body is an isolated, autonomous entity or a part of something far more interconnected. Such considerations may inspire trepidation, awe, or both, as they highlight the complexity and interconnectedness of divine creation. Alternatively, such a view can render the body ordinary or even undignified, stripping it of its unique significance within the cosmic cycle.

The Ship of Theseus is a classic thought experiment that illustrates the difficulty of these philosophical questions. It derives from an ancient Greek legend in which the ship of the hero Theseus is preserved in a harbor as a memorial. Over time, the wooden planks of the ship begin to rot, and one by one, each is replaced by a new plank. The central

38   Adam Schulman, "Wholes and Parts: Quantum Physics, Aristotelian Physics, and Environmentalism." (As cited in Kass, *The Hungry Soul*, 40.).
39   Psalm 144:4

question becomes: is it still the same ship when all the parts have been replaced?

To resolve this philosophical dilemma, Leon Kass distinguishes between two important concepts: *material* and *form*. Everything that exists, the body included, both *is* something and is *made of* something; the former is known as its form and the latter is known as its material.

As Kass suggests, "Form *is* the something made of certain materials; materials are, as materials, materials *of* and *for* the thing as formed."[40]

Bricks are simply bricks, but they become the material of a house when assembled as such by a craftsman. In this case, while the bricks retain their intrinsic properties, they are, as Kass asserts, "transformed and altered by their subordination to the activity of 'information.'"[41]

Similarly, our DNA is made of nitrogenous bases held together by alternating sugar and phosphate groups—relatively simple building blocks that can attach to each other in such a way as to form a double helix structure. But while the DNA molecule is merely material, the information it carries is far from it. Just as a written word has a visible form—a collection of letters on paper—its meaning, or the idea expressed in the word, is invisible but no less real. One of the major challenges for materialist scientists is the notion that information, which arranges parts—whether letters, wooden planks, or nucleotide bases—into a functional whole, has been consistently and repeatedly observed to be the product of intelligence, which is not material. "Form" is both the source and the result of this ordered material. Simply put, the form of the human body is its self-organizing principle.

While our material changes daily, our form—the whole—lives on. Estimates of the turnover rate of our material suggest that the body is completely renewed every 5–10 years or so. Yet our personhood remains continuous. As Kass suggests, "True, the organism is, always, coincident with its materials at any moment, but it is independent of—not tied to—any one collection of stuff over time."[42]

---

40 Kass, *The Hungry Soul.*
41 Ibid.
42 Ibid.

The ship of Theseus, according to Kass, is the same ship, just as our bodies, though constantly being remade of different stuff, are the same bodies. Indeed, it is precisely because we are constantly replacing our material that we are able to persist as beings at all. This is the achievement of form, the hallmark of which is "to keep the enmattered organization-in-action (that is, itself) both organizing and acting."[43]

A proper anthropology holds that the body is the manifestation of the person in time and space, making the invisible visible. It is also constructed to reveal what it means to be human, to reveal truths about God, our relationship to Him, and His purposes for us. The distinction between the body's material and its form—both very real and important parts of our being—contributes significantly to this revelation.

There is an aspect of our bodies—our form—that suggests that we are self-contained, distinct, and whole beings, or that we cannot be reduced to the sum of our parts. This principle, when extended to the concept of personhood, reflects not only our inherent unity as body, mind, and spirit, but also our nature as dignified individuals. Likewise, each person of the Holy Trinity—Father, Son, and Holy Spirit—is equal in divinity and retains a distinct wholeness, or a unique glory separate from the others.

Nevertheless, another aspect of our bodies—our material—teaches us that we're not entirely separate from the rest of creation. Our connection to the world and to other creatures—plant, animal, and human—is deeply ingrained in our tissues. As beings created in God's image and likeness, this characteristic finds its parallel in the communion of self-offering love among the three persons of our triune God.

But unlike the divine, who needs nothing, our needy bodies are made of the same stuff as the rest of creation and are wholly reliant on it for sustenance. If we understand creation as a manifestation of God's self-offering love, then our constant need to be fed and nourished is an object lesson in the daily need to be filled with and transformed by

---

43   Ibid.

God's love, by which we are sanctified into the kind of people who are able to offer themselves as gifts.

The Body, Redefined

Much of our discussion so far has been devoted to the human person, especially the body. We have explored its relationship to the person, its composition, and how these insights enhance our understanding of God's intentions for our embodied existence. The New Testament, however, introduces a new interpretation of the term "body" that builds on these themes. The apostle Paul employs this meaning extensively in his letters, such as in his letter to the Romans:

> "For as in one body we have many members, and the members do not all have the same function, so we, though many, are one body in Christ, and individually members one of another." (Rom. 12:4–5)

In this case, the term "body" refers to the Church, the unified body of believers with Christ as its head. This is possible because the Church is the bride of Christ, with whom He is united in one flesh. While this may be a strange and mysterious concept, it's important to recognize that Paul's choice of this term simply points to the logical conclusion of a theology of the body. In developing the purpose of the body as a visible manifestation of the person and a vessel through which our self-giving communion can be most fully expressed, the use of the term "body" in describing the Church is an appropriate way to describe the organic unity and communion between Christ and believers.

The resurrected body that Jesus presented to His followers is the redeemed body, an integral part of the person whose perfect self-mastery and sinless life allowed His body to fully express His humanity. Through the Holy Spirit, believers are called to bear the fruit of the Spirit by which we participate in this redeemed body.

But this is not the only mystery surrounding the redeemed body of Christ; this body is also the new "temple."

In the Old Testament, the temple was the dwelling place of God on earth, a gateway to heaven that allowed the people of Israel to encounter God and participate in His divine life through assembly, petition, offerings, and purification.[44]

For Jesus, the temple was His Father's house—a sacred space meant for worship, not commerce. So when He found money changers defiling it at Passover, He overturned their tables and declared, "Do not make my Father's house a house of trade" (Jn. 2:16). Outraged, the religious leaders demanded a sign of His authority. Jesus replied, "Destroy this temple, and in three days I will raise it up" (Jn. 2:19).

Jesus, of course, wasn't talking about reconstructing Herod's grand temple, the architectural wonder of Jerusalem. Rather, as John explains, Jesus was referring to His own body—a temple not built by human hands, but one that would be torn down and raised again on the third day.

A seemingly small detail solidifies this connection. At the moment of Jesus's death, the thick veil in the Jerusalem temple—the very barrier that separated the Holy of Holies from the people—was torn in two from top to bottom. What had once been an exclusive space, accessible only to the high priest, was now open to all. Through the body of Jesus, broken on the cross, believers now "have confidence to enter the holy places" (Heb. 10:19).

This confirms that, indeed, the redeemed body that was raised on the third day is the true and living temple.[45] And remarkably, those who are baptized into His body share in this temple. That's right. We, too, become a dwelling place for the presence of God to the extent that we are grafted onto His body in fellowship with His Church. As Paul reminds us, "Your body is a temple of the Holy Spirit" (1 Cor. 6:19). Through Christ, our very bodies are transformed into sacred spaces, living vessels of His divine presence.

---

44 Exodus 29:42-46.
45 Colossians 1:19

This idea is often flattened into a wellness slogan, as though Paul were merely urging believers to exercise and eat a few more fruits and vegetables so the Holy Spirit can reside in a well-toned "dream home." Contemporary talk of "temple care" that equates spa days with sanctification illustrates the point. Such a reading, however, misses Paul's larger purpose. In context, he confronts a creeping dualism that treated the body as morally irrelevant and instead affirms the believer's sacred identity through union with Christ's body. Viewed through this richer lens, genuine parallels emerge between the temple image and the way nutrition shapes embodied worship.

The Old Testament meticulously records God's specifications for the tabernacle and, later, Solomon's temple—a testament to the care and precision He required of the Israelites in constructing a place of worship. Yet these structures were merely provisional, pointing beyond themselves to something greater and more enduring: the temple of Christ's own body and, by extension, the collective body of His bride. If such detailed attention was given to temporary sanctuaries, how much more must God care about the way human bodies—the living stones of the true temple—are formed, nourished, and sustained?

As we will see, God continues to build and rebuild this temple, uniting it to Christ and nourishing the whole person—materially and spiritually—through the gift of food. A theology of food, then, becomes the next cornerstone in a Christian vision of nutrition.

2

Old Manna
(An Old Testament
Theology of Food)

Yet he commanded the skies above
and opened the doors of heaven,

and he rained down on them manna to
eat and gave them the grain of heaven.

Man ate of the bread of the angels;
he sent them food in abundance.

He caused the east wind to blow in the heavens,

and by his power he led out the south wind;

he rained meat on them like dust, winged
birds like the sand of the seas;

he let them fall in the midst of their
camp, all around their dwellings.

And they ate and were well filled, for
he gave them what they craved.

— PSALM 78:23–29

I n the last chapter, we found that the body is a manifestation of the person in time and space, making otherwise invisible realities visible. Physical hunger, then, is a design feature through which the body manifests the dependence of the whole person on the Creator. Food, when understood and received theologically, is a physical, daily reminder of this reality.

Scripture develops this theme with stories about the original diet of the nomadic Jewish tribes. This food, called "manna" and elsewhere described as the "Bread of Angels," was the staple of their forty-year journey in the wilderness and is recounted in the Book of Numbers:

> Now the manna was like coriander seed, and its appearance like that of bdellium. The people went about and gathered it and ground it in handmills or beat it in mortars and boiled it in pots and made cakes of it. And the taste of it was like the taste of cakes baked with oil. When the dew fell upon the camp in the night, the manna fell with it. (Num. 11:7–9)

Each morning, the Israelites gathered their daily portion from the ground, with a double portion on the sixth day in preparation for the Sabbath. While the details of its actual taste and texture are somewhat hazy, we can at least infer that it resembled a flaky, frosty substance that covered the ground and, when baked into cakes, had a mild sweetness and honey flavor, a foretaste of the promised land that was said to be flowing with milk and honey. This manna could not be stored; it spoiled in the sun and overnight, requiring a daily harvest—a poignant reminder of their daily dependence on God's provision.

God provided His people with a daily supply of nutritious manna, literally covering the ground for them to gather each morning—yet, dissatisfied, they grew weary of it and demanded meat. When God obliged, He brought forth a great wind from the sea and sent a huge flock of quail to fall near the camp. The people, however, gathered the quail in excess for two days and gorged themselves on the meat. Instead of simply enjoying God's provision, they acted with gluttonous disregard, revealing hearts of mistrust and ingratitude. In response to this distortion of His gift, God sent a severe plague that struck down many of the people. As Psalm 106:15 suggests, God "gave them their request; but sent leanness into their soul" (NKJV), emphasizing that when physical desires take precedence over gratitude and trust, they can lead to spiritual impoverishment.

The account of the wandering tribes in the book of Numbers highlights two timeless truths: God lovingly and abundantly provides for our needs, and we tend to resist receiving that provision as an act of grace. For forty years, God fed His people with manna, teaching them to rely on His daily gift of life—their "daily bread." Yet despite the hardships of slavery, the Israelites often looked back with longing to their former captivity in Egypt. There, they had a more varied supply of food—vegetables, fish, and occasionally meat (Num. 11:4–5)—which they recalled fondly. But their longing for Egypt stemmed not only from hunger but also from a desire for the familiarity and predictability that bondage provided, which they found easier than the wilderness journey that required trust and cultivated true freedom. With manna, God invited the Israelites into a trusting relationship defined by dependence on *His* provision rather than the security of their former bondage.

Manna is one of the most remarkable foods in the Old Testament, yet it is only one example of how food plays a crucial role in God's redemptive plan. In this exploration of Old Testament food-related themes, we will also examine the Mosaic dietary laws and the institution of sacrificial offerings. Both extend the themes introduced by the Bread of Angels but also add new dimensions to our understanding of food, one of the most tangible and relatable object lessons in the spiritual truths revealed by Christ, the true source of nourishment.

The Mosaic Dietary Law

The often-overlooked good news of the New Covenant is bacon. Picture this: for roughly 1500 years in Israel, pork, shrimp, crab, and oysters were strictly off the menu. These foods were forbidden under the dietary laws of Moses—rules many people are at least vaguely familiar with. Leviticus 11 outlines seemingly odd distinctions about land animals that "chew the cud" or "part the hoof," sea creatures that have fins and scales, insects with a certain number of legs, and so forth. By these criteria, certain creatures were declared either clean or unclean—fit for consumption or detestable.

These Old Covenant dietary regulations are among the most detailed dietary guidelines in the Bible. Their modern relevance, however, is a topic of debate. Few Christians dispute that the New Testament teaches these laws are no longer mandated; Hebrews 8:13, for example, refers to the entirety of the Old Covenant—dietary laws and all—as "obsolete." Still, many wonder if there is enduring wisdom in these Old Testament directives, making it worth voluntarily adhering to them today.

How do we approach these laws in a way that is relevant in a modern theology of food?

The Purpose of the Dietary Laws

According to Jordan Rubin, the founder of the popular "Maker's Diet," the Mosaic dietary laws remain a helpful guide for making food choices, even if they are no longer a strict requirement. Rubin suggests that dismissing them as "outdated legalism" overlooks their original intent: "to save [God's] people from physical devastation long before scientific principles of hygiene, viral transmission, bacterial infection, or molecular cell physiology were understood."[46]

Given pigs' propensity to wallow in filth and transmit trichinosis, he may have a point. If these laws reflected deep-seated natural principles of health that showcased God's foresight in preserving His people, why wouldn't health-conscious Christians consider following them voluntarily?

This logic is bolstered by the unquestioned practical utility of the ancient Jewish hygiene laws, a counterpart to the dietary laws, which undoubtedly helped the Jews fare better than their contemporaries

---

46   Jordan Rubin, *The Maker's Diet: The 40-Day Health Experience That Will Change Your Life Forever*, rev. ed. (Lake Mary, FL: Siloam Press, 2013).

during several notable plagues, such as the bubonic plague, which wiped out nearly half the population of England over the course of 250 years. As public health advocate Michael Jacobson explains, Jewish sanitation practices—outlined in Scripture centuries before the discovery of bacteria—effectively shielded them from the deadly yersinia pestis microbe.[47]

But if preventing disease and promoting health were truly the primary purposes behind these dietary and cleanliness laws, why did they cease to be promoted under the New Covenant?

Certain elements of the Mosaic Law—most notably the Ten Commandments—are reaffirmed in the New Testament, not as binding components of the old covenant, but as enduring expressions of God's unchanging moral nature. Jesus summarized their essence in the two great commandments: to love God and to love one's neighbor as oneself. These laws persist under the New Covenant, not as decrees written on stone tablets, but as inward realities written on the hearts of believers.[48]

By contrast, dietary restrictions receive no such reaffirmation. The apostle Paul even goes as far as to describe the imposition of religious dietary regulations as "the teaching of demons" (1 Tim. 4:1–3).

Mark's Gospel underscores this pivotal shift by recording Jesus's revolutionary teaching in response to criticism from the Pharisees and scribes. They had accused His disciples of breaking the traditions of the elders by eating with unwashed hands, focusing on external rituals rather than inward holiness. Addressing their misguided priorities, Jesus challenged the belief that purity depends on ritual hand washings or dietary restrictions:

> "Do you not see that whatever goes into a person from outside cannot defile him, since it enters not his heart but his stomach,

---

47   Michael F. Jacobson, *The Word on Health: A Biblical and Medical Overview of How to Care for Your Body*, rev. ed. (Washington, DC: Center for Science in the Public Interest, 2000), 45. (as cited in Rubin, *The Maker's Diet*).

48   Matthew 19:16–19; Mark 10:17–19; Luke 18:18–20.

and is expelled?" (Thus he declared all foods clean.) (Mk. 7:18–19)[49]

The parenthetical addition, "Thus he declared all foods clean," is an editorial comment by Mark that summarizes the theological implication of Jesus's teaching.[50] It's important to recognize that Jesus was not explicitly addressing clean and unclean foods, which He Himself observed under the Law. Rather, His immediate aim was to expose and discredit the traditions of the elders—human regulations that had been elevated to divine status—and to redirect attention to the true source of defilement: the condition of the heart. Mark's later interpretive comment, however, perceives in this moment a decisive turning point. In light of Christ's fulfillment of the Law, the notion of food "cleanliness" is rendered obsolete as well.

Paul also confirms this conclusion in Romans 14, writing, "I know and am persuaded in the Lord Jesus that nothing is unclean in itself," later adding, "everything is indeed clean" (Rom. 14:14, 20). This sentiment is characteristic of the entire New Testament witness: foods once deemed unclean are now "clean" in Christ.[51]

If, as many suggest, we begin with the assumption that God's Old Covenant dietary laws were given primarily for health reasons—that "clean" and "unclean" referred to biological realities—then the New Testament's clear and consistent teaching that all foods are now clean would leave us with only one conclusion: that God altered the laws of nature. Of course, this conclusion is dubious, at best. There is no indication that Jesus tampered with any natural realities; He didn't

---

49 This point, if taken to its logical conclusion, seems to push back against the notion that our food becomes a part of us, a scientific reality that is unquestioned and which has philosophical implications that we've already begun to explore. Yet this teaching, spoken in simple terms that even a child could understand, is not a commentary on digestion, but is intended to point to a deeper truth about spiritual defilement.

50 Some have argued that the phrase "thus he declared all foods clean" is a mistranslation of the original Greek, which more literally reads "cleansing all foods." They suggest that Jesus was merely referring to the body's natural digestive process rather than making a theological statement about dietary laws. However, this interpretation is strained both grammatically and contextually.

51 1 Timothy 4:3–5; Titus 1:14-15; Colossians 2:16–17, 20–22; Hebrews 9:9–10, 13:9

implore pigs to clean up their act, nor did He change any intrinsic truths about disease transmission. The more reasonable conclusion, then, is that our initial assumption is mistaken. The dietary laws must have served a different purpose that found its fulfillment in Christ.

John Calvin, in his commentary on Leviticus, is emphatic that Moses was not acting as God's public health official. He writes, "Those who imagine that God here had regard to their health, as if discharging the office of a Physician, pervert by their vain speculation the whole force and utility of this law."[52] Instead, Calvin argues, these regulations served a distinct and temporary purpose for a specific people at a particular time in redemptive history.

But while these laws were never meant to serve as a textbook on nutrition, they offer profound insights into the character of God and His intentions for His chosen people. In short, the laws themselves may be obsolete, but their modern-day implications are far from it. Before we explore these implications, however, it's important to consider how these laws have been historically understood, especially as we look back from the privileged vantage point of Christianity.

First and foremost, the dietary laws were established to set God's people apart, ensuring they would be distinct among the nations and protected from the corrupting influences of neighboring pagan cultures. As Thomas Aquinas put it, the laws helped "withdraw the people from the fellowship of idolators."[53]

This temporary purpose is evident in Leviticus 11, which does not classify animals as inherently "clean" or "unclean" in a universal sense, but rather as ones *"you* may eat" versus those that are "unclean *to you."* The phrase "to you" makes it clear that these rules were specifically tailored for Israel, serving as a covenantal sign rather than a statement about the animals' intrinsic nature.

A similar emphasis on separation appears in Leviticus 20:24–26:

---

52 John Calvin, Commentaries on the Four Last Books of Moses, trans. Charles William Bingham (Grand Rapids: Eerdmans, 1950), 3:372.

53 Thomas Aquinas, Summa Theologiae, I–II, q. 102, a. 6.

"I am the LORD your God, who has separated you from the peoples. You shall therefore separate the clean beast from the unclean, and the unclean bird from the clean. You shall not make yourselves detestable by beast or by bird or by anything with which the ground crawls, which I have set apart for you to hold unclean. You shall be holy to me, for I the LORD am holy and have separated you from the peoples, that you should be mine."

The fact that the unique diet of the Jews was intended to have such a profoundly segregating effect illustrates a fundamental truth: Eating fosters communion with others. Shared meals are uniquely emblematic of fellowship, breaking down barriers, reinforcing a shared human neediness, and promoting genuine hospitality. They shape rituals, norms, and values. Eating together, an act that precedes and helps forge deeper social bonds, is the stepping stone to marrying together, which could have compromised Israel's redemptive mission as a people set apart by God.

But God didn't just want His people to be distinct among the nations; He wanted them to be distinct *and holy*—a living testimony to their loving and sustaining Creator. Here, the law—described by Paul as a teacher—used food not only to cultivate obedience, but also to develop in the Israelites a sharpened discernment for what is pleasing to the Lord.

This purpose is clearly stated in Leviticus 10:10: "You are to distinguish between the holy and the common, and between the unclean and the clean." This conveys the broader idea that human nature finds its fullest expression in discerning the virtuous, beautiful, and pure from the sinful, detestable, and defiled.

Leon Kass observes that "the first reason for the dietary laws is the need to restrain, moderate, and define the naturally unrestrained, immoderate, and boundless appetites of human beings—appetites that are by no means restricted to the desires for food but for which the problem of eating is somehow emblematic."[54]

---

54   Much of the following discussion on the symbolism of the dietary laws is adapted from Leon R. Kass, "Why the Dietary Laws?" *Commentary Magazine*, September 3, 2015.

In this view, learning to distinguish among foods is merely the first step in learning to govern all human desires. By developing a disciplined approach to eating, the Jewish people were distinguishing themselves not only as a people set apart, but as a *righteous* people set apart by a *holy* God.

Peter's Vision: The Sheet from Heaven (Acts 10:9–16)

While praying on a rooftop, Peter sees a vision of a sheet descending from heaven, filled with all kinds of animals—both clean and unclean. A voice from heaven commands, "Rise, Peter; kill and eat." Peter protests, saying he has never eaten anything unclean. The voice replies, "What God has made clean, do not call common." This exchange occurs three times for emphasis.

Though the vision prepares Peter to welcome Gentiles into the covenant community, its symbolism is anchored in the categories of clean and unclean foods. It is not merely about people; it's about the fulfillment of the entire clean/unclean system in Christ. The key to understanding this vision lies in Peter's personal struggle: a lifelong observant Jew, his deep-seated reluctance shows how difficult it was to accept that these laws had been fulfilled. But this is likely the moment in which Jesus's teachings finally sunk in.

Importantly, Peter is understood to be the primary informant behind Mark's Gospel. In both accounts (Mark 7 and Acts 10), the same Greek terms for "cleanse" (katharizō) and "defile" (koinoō) are used in direct contrast, showing a deliberate connection. What Jesus taught during His earthly ministry, Peter now grasps through divine revelation. The vision confirms that the food laws were never about health, but about symbolic holiness, obedience, and covenantal separation—temporary shadows pointing to the substance found in Christ.

In Him, that purpose is fulfilled, and alligator burgers and vulture stew are back on the menu!

The Symbolism of the Dietary Laws

Having established that the primary purpose of the dietary laws was to set God's people apart as a holy nation, preserved to carry God's promise to its fulfillment in Jesus, the choice of which animals were deemed clean or unclean could well have been arbitrary and still achieved this goal. It seems, however, that there was a symbolic meaning to these distinctions—one that likely reinforced the overarching theme of separation by echoing the divisions established in God's creation.

The dietary laws served as a continual reminder that God is a God of order, creating distinctions with divine purpose. By adhering to a meaningful set of dietary distinctions, the Israelites mirrored God's creative work and participated in His likeness, aligning themselves with His divine logic and affirming their role as a people set apart.

The theme of order goes back to Genesis, where God creates distinct categories of animals with purposeful boundaries according to a classification system that differs greatly from our modern view of the animal kingdom. Rather than grouping animals based on biological characteristic and in classes such as mammals, reptiles, and invertebrates, Scripture generally sorts them by their habitat and relationship to it— land animals, sea creatures, and flying things.[55] For example, in this ancient classification system, dolphins (which modern biology considers to be mammals) are lumped together with the fish as sea creatures.

The dietary laws had unique cleanliness requirements for each of these categories:

Land Animals. Among the land animals, only those that both "part the hoof" and "chew the cud" were considered clean.[56] This criterion allowed for ruminants (e.g., cattle, sheep, goats, and deer) but

---

55   Genesis 1:25. Within the land animals there are further subdivisions (beasts of the earth, livestock, and creeping things). Again, these subdivisions are based on distinctions in the environment. The livestock live near man, the beasts of the earth are distant (in the wilderness), and the creeping things tend to be undesirable animals that live alongside man, such as rodents and snakes.

56   "Chewing the cud" referred to ruminants, or what Kass calls "chew chewers"—animals with multiple stomachs that regurgitate and rechew partially digested food.

excluded pigs (cloven-footed but non-ruminant) and camels (ruminant but without cloven hooves). Animals that walk on paws or swarm on the ground were deemed unclean.

Sea Creatures. The aquatic animals were clean only if they had both scales and fins, which excluded shellfish, catfish, and eels, for example.

Flying Things. The Israelites were given only a short list of unclean birds, generally scavengers and birds of prey (e.g., eagles, vultures, and owls), while birds such as chickens, turkeys, and ducks were permitted.

Winged Insects. Only those with jointed legs (e.g., locusts, crickets, and grasshoppers) were considered clean.

Scripture doesn't specify the symbolic meaning underlying these distinctions, so any attempt to assign meaning is speculative. Nevertheless, certain notable themes emerge. Kass observes that, just as the dietary laws were intended to set a people apart from their neighbors, clean animals generally reflect the divisions within God's created order, whereas unclean animals often blur those boundaries.

Consider the exclusion of amphibians, which have no proper place either in the water or on land. Also deemed unclean were creatures lacking a proper form: those with fluid forms lacking a true boundary (e.g., sea creatures without scales); those with deceptive forms (e.g., eels and other fish that don't resemble typical fish); and those with incomplete forms (e.g., land animals with incompletely cloven hooves).

Animals without a means of locomotion suited to their form or environment were also excluded. Examples include sea creatures that walk on the ground like land animals (e.g., crabs and lobsters); land animals that swarm on the ground as though moving through water (e.g., snakes); and those that walk on paws, essentially using their hands for feet (e.g., dogs and cats).

Finally, the diets of the animals played a significant role. Ruminants, which chew the cud, exemplify a "pure" diet, ensuring that Jews could not indirectly violate the dietary laws by consuming animals that fed on impure substances. This principle is reinforced by the exclusion of carnivores and scavengers, whose feeding habits are fundamentally at odds with the idea of purity.[57]

By following these dietary laws, Israel "paid homage to the articulated order of the world and the dignity of life and living form … and they celebrated, in gratitude and reverence, the mysterious source of the articulated world and its generous hospitality in providing food, both for life and for thought."[58]

In summary, God used the Mosaic dietary laws to set apart a holy people by teaching them to distinguish between clean and unclean. At first, these rules may appear arbitrary, but closer examination reveals a pattern of divine order symbolized by the animals themselves.

When Jesus declared all foods clean, He didn't change any fundamental scientific truths, because the laws were never meant to reveal timeless health and wellness principles. Rather, He transformed the covenantal context: the distinctions between Jew and Gentile were dissolved in Him. By fully embodying the obedience, holiness, and covenantal separation that the dietary laws expressed and affected, Jesus brought them to their intended fulfillment. But while the laws themselves are now obsolete and have no need of being resurrected, their underlying message remains: God's people are still called to live— and eat—with distinctiveness. The Christian diet may not have food rules, but that doesn't mean there isn't a uniquely Christian approach to nutrition that we are called to uphold. We'll continue laying the foundation for that approach by examining another relevant aspect of the law that Jesus fulfilled on the cross.

Sacrifice

Just as the Old Covenant mandated special dietary restrictions, it also featured laws of sacrifice. The presentation of sacrificial offerings was central to Israelite culture, continuing until the destruction of the

---

57 Kass, "Why the Dietary Laws?"
58 Ibid.

temple in 70 AD. These sacrifices served several symbolic purposes: they promoted humility before God, fostered a trusting dependence on the source of all good gifts, and offered a debt when those gifts were perverted by sin. If the dietary laws conveyed the lesson that our food choices have effects that reach into the very fabric of our personhood, the demands of ritual worship added a parallel lesson about giving and receiving the gift of self.

While there were a number of specific sacrifices for various occasions, they fell into two main categories: bloody and unbloody.

Bloody, or *propitiatory*, sacrifices focused on atonement, allowing repentant sinners to transfer the consequences of sin to an unblemished substitute. Because an animal's life resides in its blood, the spilling of blood was essential for a substitute worthy of taking one's place.[59]

At its core, such a sacrifice could paradoxically be thought of as a "gift of self." By placing a prized animal on the altar, the worshiper offered not only the resources and care invested in raising the animal, but food that would have been converted into material for his own body. As the Swiss theologian Karl Barth explains, "When he destroys the animal and sheds its blood ... he renounces its use for his own sustenance and enjoyment and surrenders it to God as a representation of that which God in His grace really is for him."[60] This act involved a kind of death—a temporary loss of one's sustenance in exchange for a visceral recognition of the true source of life. Bloody sacrifice was a somber reminder that death produces new life.

The principle is evident in nature. Soil, for example, comes alive through the decomposition of countless organisms—plants, animals, and microbes—all of which contribute to the fertility that spawns more life. Human beings are formed out of dirt—out of this death—as both our origin story and our daily experience of eating plants and animals attest.

This physical reality mirrors a deeper spiritual one. In John 12:24, Jesus teaches, "Truly, truly, I say to you, unless a grain of wheat falls into

---

59   Leviticus 17:11

60   Karl Barth, *Church Dogmatics, The Doctrine of Creation*, vol. 3, part 4, trans. G. W. Bromiley and R. J. Ehrlich (Edinburgh: T&T Clark, 2000), 324.

the earth and dies, it remains alone; but if it dies, it bears much fruit." All of Scripture describes the need to die in order to be transformed into a new fullness of life. This death that breeds life—a death in which the person gives not only the product of his labor, but a small part of himself—is the means by which one is transformed into the type of person who is capable of receiving the gift of creation.

Not all sacrifices required bloodshed, however. A second broad category, the "unbloody" sacrifices, involved presenting a small share of one's bounty back to its ultimate source in thanksgiving rather than atonement. While animal sacrifices are much more commonly associated with ancient Israel, unbloody offerings were no less important or prevalent.

Among the unbloody offerings, the "bread of the Presence"—also called "showbread"—may be unfamiliar to many modern Christians. It is rarely mentioned in Scripture, tucked away in long passages of Exodus that meticulously describe the construction of the tabernacle, the mobile precursor to the Temple in Jerusalem. But this bread was a big deal to the ancient Jews. In fact, it was one of only three items reserved for the Holy Place of the tabernacle, alongside the golden lampstand (menorah) and the altar of incense.

Each Sabbath, the priests baked twelve loaves of bread—representing the twelve tribes of Israel—and offered them with wine on a table made of acacia wood and overlaid with pure gold. This bread and wine symbolized two key realities. First, because the bread remained continually before God, with the menorah always lit, it represented God's enduring presence. Second, it served as a sign of God's covenant with Israel, much like to a wedding ring signifying an enduring family bond.[61]

Make no mistake, however, the bread of the Presence wasn't just a symbol; it was an offering. Exodus 25 stipulates that incense—used for sacrifices—be placed beside the showbread, indicating the rising fragrance of worship.[62] When this offering was replaced each Sabbath

---

61   Leviticus 24:8

62   The prophet Ezekiel bolsters this claim by referring to the table of the bread of the Presence as an "altar" in Ezekiel 41:21-22.

day, the old bread became a meal for the priests, symbolizing the meal enjoyed by Moses and the elders of Israel when they saw the face of God on Mt. Sinai.[63] In other words, as Brant Pitre explains, "It was both a gift from God to his priests (in the form of a meal) and an offering of the priests to their God (in the form of a sacrifice)."[64]

The idea that the bread of the Presence symbolized Moses's encounter with the "face" of God is far from trivial. In Hebrew, the word for "presence" is *panim*, meaning "face."[65] Therefore, the bread of the Presence was also called the "bread of the face." This detail is striking in light of the Old Covenant command for all Jewish men to "appear before the Lord" three times a year.

Exodus 34:23 reads, "Three times in the year shall all your males appear before the Lord God, the God of Israel," but in Hebrew it literally says, "Three times a year shall all your males see the face of the Lord," using the same word *panim* found in "bread of the face."[66]

So how did Jewish men fulfill this command? According to first-century sources, the priests in the Jerusalem Temple would unveil the bread of the Presence and hold it aloft before the pilgrims, proclaiming, "Behold, God's love for you!"[67]

Aside from the remarkable choice of food as a symbol of God's love for His people, we are faced with a perplexing question: Why did God choose mere loaves of bread for His earthly image—His "face"? For some reason, bread appears again and again in the Old Testament as the embodiment of human nourishment, but why? Before we answer that question, let us first consider the significance of bread.

---

63   Exodus 24 and 29.

64   Brant Pitre, *Jesus and the Jewish Roots of the Eucharist* (New York: Image, 2011).

65   Ibid., 121.

66   Pitre, *Jesus and the Jewish Roots of the Eucharist*, 132.

67   Babylonian Talmud, Menahoth 29A (As cited in Pitre, *Jesus and the Jewish Roots of the Eucharist*, 131).

Why Bread?

The Paleolithic, or "Paleo," diet regards agriculture as one of history's most regrettable innovations. Also known as the Caveman, Stone Age, or Steak and Bacon Diet, it claims that eating like our most primitive ancestors aligns with our genetics and promotes robust health. Anything that can be hunted, fished, or gathered is allowed, but grains, legumes, and dairy are off-limits because they are believed to underlie many of the health problems that afflict modern humans.

We need not dismiss this claim outright, for one could do much worse than a diet based on these whole, minimally processed staples. But the notion that we can—and should—revert to a romanticized "golden age," free from society's trappings, is a fallacy as old as civilization itself.

This nostalgia for pre-agrarian life resonates with the earliest biblical depiction of humanity's self-understanding, in which bread, the staple of the human diet, is closely tied to the Fall. In Genesis 3, God says to Adam,

> "Cursed is the ground because of you; in pain you shall eat of it all the days of your life; thorns and thistles it shall bring forth for you; and you shall eat the plants of the field. By the sweat of your face you shall eat bread, till you return to the ground ..." (Gen. 3:17–19)

Love it or hate it, bread is the quintessential human food—especially in our fallen condition. It represents the transition from gathering abundant fruit in Eden to laboring for sustenance. The craft of breadmaking, in Kass's words, "involves artfully overcoming the natural incapacity for digesting grain," an endeavor that "both requires and effects massive transformations in the human way of life."[68]

This innovation spurred the need for agriculture—plowing, sowing, harvesting, and storing—and eventually for crafts such as metalworking and animal husbandry. Agriculture demanded planning, delayed gratification, and reliance on God for the harvest. It required

---

68   Kass, *The Hungry Soul*, 121.

settlement in one place, fostered a sense of responsibility for one's labor and for the soil itself, and grounded the concepts of personal property and justice.

As Kass succinctly puts it, "A transformer of nature, a practitioner of art, a restrainer of his own appetites, a settled social creature soon with laws and rules of justice, poised proudly yet apprehensively between the earth and the cosmic powers—man becomes human with the eating of bread."[69]

Some people see this bread-fueled development of civilization as a downfall—humanity's root corruption. Christians, however, should see it differently. It was not bread that corrupted mankind, but original sin. The so-called "curse" of bread may be part of God's loving plan to cultivate an ordered, just, and distinctly human society in a world of toil and effort.

Indeed, the connection between bread and human life is powerfully affirmed in Deuteronomy 24:6, where the law explicitly forbids taking a millstone—even just the upper millstone—as collateral for a debt. To do so, the text says, would be equivalent to "taking a life in pledge." In ancient Israel, bread was so essential to survival that depriving someone of the means to make it was equivalent to depriving them of life itself. Bread, in this sense, is not just food—it is a symbol of human vulnerability, labor, and dignity. Only with this context in mind can our modern ears grasp why bread so powerfully symbolizes human nourishment.

Given bread's distinct anthropological role, the bread of the Presence was hardly an arbitrary offering. Nor was it something novel or unprecedented. Long before the Old Covenant was established, bread and wine were already being offered to God—as a symbol of human nourishment and, therefore, a symbol of self.

---

69   Ibid., 122.

Melchizedek

In the book of Genesis, not long after the Flood, we encounter a mysterious figure who is mentioned only briefly in the Old Testament. He appears in Genesis 14, following Abraham's victory over several pagan kings in his mission to rescue his nephew, Lot. As Abraham returns from battle, he is met by Melchizedek, described as both king of Salem and priest of God Most High:

> After his return from the defeat of Chedorlaomer and the kings who were with him, the king of Sodom went out to meet him at the Valley of Shaveh (that is, the King's Valley). And Melchizedek king of Salem brought out bread and wine. (He was priest of God Most High.) And he blessed him and said, "Blessed be Abram by God Most High, Possessor of heaven and earth; and blessed be God Most High, who has delivered your enemies into your hand! And Abram gave him a tenth of everything." (Gen. 14:17–20)

Who is this man to whom Abraham—Israel's great patriarch— voluntarily offered a tenth of his spoils?[70] Genesis identifies Melchizedek as both king of Salem (likely the precursor to Jerusalem) and priest of God Most High. His name translates as "king of righteousness," pointing to a status beyond that of an ordinary priest or king. The writer of Hebrews later stresses that Melchizedek outranked Abraham, implying a superior priesthood to that of Levi, who was "in the loins" of Abraham at the time (Heb. 7:2–10).

Melchizedek, a king-priest whose greatness surpassed even that of Abraham, Aaron, and the Levitical priesthood, served as a "type" of Christ—a Christ-like forerunner pointing to Jesus, the true and ultimate High Priest.

---

70 This original tithe (one-tenth offering) was from Abraham, 400 years before the Law of Moses.

Hundreds of years before God instituted the bread of the Presence, Melchizedek offered the Lord not meat, but bread and wine! In Jewish tradition, this act is sometimes seen as the origin of the bread of the Presence, a ritual Melchizedek is believed to have passed on to Abraham.[71]

Therefore, while the bloody sacrifices were vital—foreshadowing the perfect, propitiatory sacrifice of Christ—we should not overlook the significance of the unbloody offerings of grain and bread. These, too, pointed forward to another divine gift: not only Christ offered *for* us, but Christ given *to* us as true food and true drink.

An Appetizer for the True "Bread of Life"

The significance of food in the Old Testament cannot be overstated. Again and again, it serves as an object lesson for countless spiritual truths that point us to Christ. In analyzing the dietary laws that set God's people apart, we indirectly learn about a meal's power to unite in fellowship and we see that our dietary choices are important to the Lord. When we recall God providing manna, we consider His abundant care for His people and are reminded of our daily dependence on Him. In sacrificial rituals, we see this offering reciprocated as a means of thanksgiving or substitutionary atonement, but always as a sign of self.

Together, these practices reveal God's plan to cultivate in His people an awareness of creation's original fullness: a simplicity in receiving His gracious gifts and transforming them into offerings of self.

If the Old Testament lays the groundwork for this theme, then Jesus stands as its ultimate fulfillment—a truth that vividly emerges in the recurring motif of bread. As the quintessential human food, bread was among humanity's earliest offerings. Over time, it came to signify God's covenant, His love, and even His image on earth.

For these reasons, God's command to house not only a jar of manna but also the bread of the Presence continually within the temple is not unexpected—yet it remains deeply significant. And though the physical

---

71   Genesis Rabbah, 43:6 (as cited in Pitre, *Jesus and the Jewish Roots of the Eucharist*, 127).

Temple no longer stands, He *still* requires these signs to be continually housed in the true Temple.

As the next chapter will show, Jesus—the great High Priest in the order of Melchizedek—offers Himself not only as the spotless sacrifice of the New Covenant but also as the living food by which its promises are continually sealed. When believers partake of this bread and wine, they are, as we saw in Chapter One, transformed into the living Temple—the body of Christ. Therefore, while Moses called down manna from heaven, Jesus is its greater fulfillment—the true "Bread of Life."

3

New Manna
(A New Testament
Theology of Food)

*"To be sure, food keeps us alive, but that is
only its smallest and most temporary work. Its
eternal purpose is to furnish our sensibilities
against the day when we shall sit down at the
heavenly banquet and see how gracious the
Lord is. Nourishment is necessary only for a
while; what we shall need forever is taste."*

*"Food is the daily sacrament of unnecessary
goodness, ordained for a continual remembrance
that the world will always be more delicious
than it is useful. Necessity is the mother only of
cliches. It takes playfulness to make poetry."*

—ROBERT FARRAR CAPON, THE SUPPER OF THE LAMB

In Hebrew, Bethlehem means "House of Bread."[72] How fitting, then, that Jesus was born in a place whose very name reflects His deep identification with food and drink. During His earthly ministry, Christ was considered a drunkard by the Pharisees, the strictest keepers of the law. Matthew describes His reputation in this way: "The Son of Man came eating and drinking, and they say, 'Look at him! A glutton and a drunkard, a friend of tax collectors and sinners!'" (Matt. 11:19).[73] Although this charge was a gross exaggeration, the Pharisees were right to notice the central role of food in Jesus's public life.

As Robert Karris observes, "In Luke's Gospel Jesus is either going to a meal, at a meal, or coming from a meal."[74] His first public miracle was turning water into wine at a wedding feast in Cana. He dined with tax collectors, sinners, and Pharisees, and He fed thousands by multiplying five loaves and two fish. After His resurrection, He even prepared breakfast for His disciples on the shore. In short, Christ used food as the centerpiece of his message of salvation, fulfilling the sacrificial altar and instituting the table in its place. He embraced the table not only for its communal potential, but also to proclaim a radical message that defied social norms. Above all, Christ used food to describe Himself, declaring that He was true, living nourishment—the fulfillment of every Old Testament signpost pointing to Him.[75]

Nowhere is this more evident than in the Gospel of John, particularly in the famous Bread of Life discourse (John 6). In this chapter, Jesus addresses a large crowd—an audience steeped in Jewish traditions and Messianic expectations. Like most first-century Jews, this

---

72   John Everett-Heath, *The Concise Dictionary of World Place-Names* (Oxford: Oxford University Press, 2005).

73   To our modern ears, the terms "glutton and drunkard" may not carry the same weight as they likely did to Matthew's contemporaries, but scholars point to two Old Testament passages that shed light on the meaning of the insult. In Deuteronomy 21:18–21, it is used in the context of purging evil from Israel, describing gluttons and drunkards as those who should be stoned to death. Likewise, Proverbs 23:20 says, "Be not among drunkards or among gluttonous eaters of meat."

74   Robert J. Karris, *Eating Your Way Through Luke's Gospel* (Collegeville, MN: Liturgical Press, 2006), 14.

75   Isaiah 55:2.

audience would have been eagerly anticipating a new Exodus, marked by four great events:

1. the arrival of a new Moses;
2. the establishment of a new covenant;
3. the construction of a new temple; and
4. the journey to a new promised land.[76]

Jesus intentionally crafted His ministry to demonstrate that these long-anticipated promises found their fulfillment in Him. Earlier in John 6, the crowd had witnessed the miraculous multiplication of the loaves and fishes, followed by Jesus walking on water—both acts deliberately evocative of the wilderness provision and Red Sea crossing under Moses. Confronted with such signs, many in the crowd would have naturally wondered, "Could this be the new Moses we have been waiting for?"

Seeking further confirmation, they pressed Jesus for another miracle, one that would mirror the daily manna their ancestors received in the wilderness. John records their request and Jesus's reply in verses 30–35:

> So they said to him, "Then what sign do you do, that we may see and believe you? What work do you perform? Our fathers ate the manna in the wilderness; as it is written, 'He gave them bread from heaven to eat.'" Jesus then said to them, "Truly, truly, I say to you, it was not Moses who gave you the bread from heaven, but my Father gives you the true bread from heaven. For the bread of God is he who comes down from heaven and gives life to the world." ... Jesus said to them, "I am the bread of life; whoever comes to me shall not hunger, and whoever believes in me shall never thirst."

---

76   Pitre, *Jesus and the Jewish Roots of the Eucharist*, 24.

The crowd, growing visibly impatient for a new outpouring of miraculous bread, much like the manna their ancestors had received, still misunderstood the sign. Jesus was offering them something far greater: a new manna, not simply to sustain physical life for a day, but to nourish them eternally.

> "Your fathers ate the manna in the wilderness, and they died. This is the bread that comes down from heaven, so that one may eat of it and not die. I am the living bread that came down from heaven. If anyone eats of this bread, he will live forever. And the bread that I will give for the life of the world is my flesh." (Jn. 6:49–51)

Understandably, this teaching continued to baffle the listeners, who were unfamiliar with the kind of eating that Jesus was talking about. "How can this man give us his flesh to eat?" (v. 52). But instead of reassuring them, Jesus intensified His language:

> "Whoever *feeds* on my flesh and *drinks* my blood has eternal life, and I will raise him up on the last day. For my flesh is true food, and my blood is true drink." (Jn. 6:54-55)

In the original Greek passage, John's word for "eat" shifts from *phagein* (a standard term) to *trógō*, meaning "gnaw" or "chew," suggesting a more deliberate, visceral action in these verses. By using such graphic language, Jesus reinforced the seriousness and depth of His message, conveying a deeper, more sustained participation.

But despite the graphic imagery, when Jesus described His flesh as the true food for the "life of the world," He was alluding to an entirely different *kind* of eating—not carnal or corporeal, but spiritual—a reality that was difficult for the assembled crowd to grasp and fundamentally different from the physical eating of manna. "The words I have spoken to you are spirit and life," He says in verse 63.

What exactly was Jesus talking about? What kind of eating is this, if not physical?

Jesus was speaking of food that requires faith not only to comprehend but also to receive—a form of nourishment mediated by the power of the Holy Spirit. But while mysterious, this kind of eating wasn't exactly new. It had long been foreshadowed in Deuteronomy 8:3, which insists that "man does not live by bread alone, but … by every word that comes from the mouth of the Lord." Physical food alone cannot sustain the whole person; true life requires ingesting the Lord's Word.

Recall, however, that the Gospel of John identifies Jesus as the eternal Word made flesh (Jn. 1), making the "Bread of Life" and "Word of God" one and the same. This Jesus is the same Word who was in the beginning with God, and who was God, through whom all things were made, and whom Deuteronomy 8:3 tells us should be a part of our diet. The superior, life-giving food alluded to in Deuteronomy is and always has been of the same kind that Jesus attributed to Himself.

While John 6 certainly points back to the Old Testament, it also points forward to the Last Supper, the culmination of a theology of food, where Jesus fulfills and redefines the long-anticipated new Exodus with a new and greater Passover.

On the night of His betrayal, Jesus gave new covenantal meaning to the traditional Passover bread and wine, commanding His disciples to find refuge under His perfect blood, just as the Israelites had once found refuge under the blood of the Passover lamb.[77] When He broke the bread, He said, "This is my body, which is for you. Do this in remembrance of me." Likewise, He took the cup and said, "This cup is the new covenant in my blood. Do this, as often as you drink it, in remembrance of me" (1 Cor. 11:24–25).

In the Lord's Supper, believers obey Christ's command and partake of the new Passover meal, renewing and sealing the promises of the New Covenant. In this act, they participate in the mysterious form of eating that once confounded Jesus's Jewish followers—a spiritual

---

77   Thomas R. Schreiner and Matthew R. Crawford, eds., *The Lord's Supper: Remembering and Proclaiming Christ until He Comes* (Nashville: B&H Publishing Group, 2011), 93.

feeding in which, by the power of the Holy Spirit, their souls are lifted to heaven to truly partake of Christ in His full humanity and divinity. This sacramental act has a sanctifying effect, as God graciously nourishes and transforms those who receive it in faith, strengthening their union with Christ, and reorienting them away from sin and toward righteousness.

If sin can be understood as a refusal to receive the world as a gift, then the Supper stands as a restorative act—opening our eyes to behold creation rightly: not as something to be consumed on our terms, but as a gift to be received and enjoyed according to God's.[78]

In short, ordinary bread and wine become, for believers, the true nourishment of Christ Himself—the sign and seal of His sustaining grace. And as Augustine beautifully put it, "If you receive them well, you are what you receive." Through this divine provision, Christ feeds His people and conforms them more fully into His likeness.

Augustine, way ahead of his time, seems to have been confirming the modern sentiment, "You are what you eat," at least when it comes to the Supper. Yet this transformation is unlike anything we experience at an ordinary table. In daily life, we consume food and turn it into more of ourselves. But in this sacred meal, the opposite occurs: it is not the body that transforms the food, but the food that transforms the body. As Martin Luther describes,

> "Perishable food is transformed into the body which eats it; this food, however, transforms the person who eats it into itself, and makes him like itself, spiritual, alive, and eternal … His flesh is … a food of an entirely different kind … and does not let itself be transformed, but transforms those who eat it, and it gives them the Spirit … It is as if a wolf devoured a sheep and the sheep were so powerful a food that it transformed the wolf and turned him into a sheep. So when we eat Christ's flesh physically and spiritually, the food is so powerful that it transforms us into

---

78   This isn't necessarily a precise description of sin, but instead is meant to highlight an aspect of sin that is particularly relevant to this discussion.

itself and out of fleshly, sinful, mortal men makes us spiritual, holy, living men."[79]

Simply put, the Lord's Supper is the summit of eating. As we observe it, we look back to the cross, we look around at the community of believers, and we look forward to the coming heavenly wedding feast, where this meal will be seen as a mere appetizer.[80] But while the sacrament is indispensable as a regular practice within the Church, it also informs us about the meaning of food in general, both fulfilling and expanding the principles developed in the Old Testament.

This point cannot be overstated: by calling Himself "true food," Jesus perfectly reveals what food is meant to be. Our bodies are most deeply nourished when they share in Christ at His table, so every other table becomes a kind of rehearsal—either of that communion or of its counterfeit. The Christian task is to eat in ways that continually recall, rehearse, and reinforce our union with the Lord who feeds us with Himself. We might call this practice "Eucharistic eating"—applying the logic of the Lord's Supper to our ordinary meals. In the pages that follow, we will develop two core themes—*thanksgiving* and *reconciliation*—as a foundational (though not exhaustive) meditation on what Eucharistic eating looks like in practice.

Thanksgiving

The richness and numerous purposes of the Lord's Supper are conveyed by the various names given to it, such as the Breaking of Bread or the Holy Communion. But of these names, "the Eucharist" best conveys its core identity as the Church's proclamation of thanksgiving. Derived from the Greek word *eucharistia* (meaning "thanksgiving" or "gratitude"), this term traces back to Jesus's words of institution when He gave thanks before offering the cup of His blood. In the Eucharist,

---

79   Martin Luther, "This is My Body," 1527 (as cited in Kleinig, *Wonderfully Made*, 84).
80   Schreiner and Crawford, *The Lord's Supper*, 44, 58.

the faithful give thanks to God not only for creation and sustenance, but also for the redemption accomplished in Jesus.

This attitude of thanksgiving applies as much to our regular meals as it does to the Eucharist. Paul stresses this in 1 Timothy 4:4–5:

> "For everything created by God is good, and nothing is to be rejected if it is received with thanksgiving, for it is made holy by the word of God and prayer."

Just as the Church gives thanks for the perfect sacrifice of its Savior, giving thanks at mealtimes is a way of demonstrating and fostering a spirit of humility before the Lord as a body in constant need of nourishment. It also reminds us that the ultimate source of our food is not our own labor, but the generous hand of the Creator, whose love is manifested as something mouthwatering on the plate. Wirzba describes food as "God's love made nutritious and delicious," and eating as "the daily reminder that life comes to us as a gift."[81] Theologian Alexander Schmemann similarly observes that God's "remembrance" of us is the gift of life, which we receive and increase through our own remembrance of Him.[82] In giving thanks, we allow the food to transform us, much as the Eucharist does, making us better able to see the world as a gift.

It's easy to forget to give thanks for our food, largely because we don't recognize it as a gift in the first place. This blindness often stems from a strained relationship with food, one shaped by a utilitarian mindset that reduces it to mere fuel.

We often treat food as a container for calories, reducible to numbers to be tallied throughout the day. This reductionist view fosters a collective impression that food is something to be guarded against, as if flavor and healthfulness occupy opposite ends of a spectrum. Rich, satisfying foods like whole milk, butter, and bacon are often blamed for weight gain and disease. Meanwhile, so-called "health foods" are

---

81   Wirzba, *Food and Faith*.

82   Alexander Schmemann, *The Eucharist* (Crestwood, NY: St. Vladimir's Seminary Press, 1988) (as cited in Wirzba, *Food and Faith*).

perceived as low-calorie, bland, and unsatisfying—a limp salad here, a dollop of low-fat yogurt there, and maybe a sprinkling of nuts.

Episcopal priest and chef Robert Farrar Capon vividly captures this tension:

"The modern diet victim sees his life at the table not as a delightful alternation between pearls of great price and dishes of lesser cost, but as a grim sentence which condemns him to pay for every fattening repast (even the sleaziest) with a meal of carrot sticks and celery. Not that there is anything wrong with raw vegetables, or with eating less if you want to—but to allow such considerations to become the rule of man's eating is simply the death of dining."[83]

Caught between indulgence and health, many find themselves in a grim paradox. Eating becomes a means to an end, and food is stripped of its inherent beauty, reduced to a sterile collection of nutrients, either "good" or "bad." In this mindset, there's little room for gratitude.

But this perspective misses something important. Food, like our bodies, is not just *made of* something; it *is* something. Food, by virtue of being food, is precious before the stuff it's made of ever becomes useful. Make no mistake: the practical consideration of assembling a diet with the right nutrients is indeed important, and will receive due attention in much of this book. But first, let's reflect on what food really is.

Let's start with a thought experiment: Imagine that utility alone was humanity's highest good—that we were intended to see things only in terms of their usefulness. If that were true, wouldn't God, in His infinite wisdom, have created a single, perfect, nutritionally complete food source for us to consume forever? This, of course, would be the optimal solution to our bodily neediness. But remember that manna was such a food source for the wandering tribes of Israel, and yet they

---

83   Robert Farrar Capon, *The Supper of the Lamb: A Culinary Reflection* (New York: Modern Library, 1989).

grumbled. A monotonous diet may satisfy physical needs, but human beings hunger for more than mere utility.

In a utilitarian world, there would be no need for onions to differ from beets. Yet God made onions distinct from beets simply because He delights in their differences. It's unnecessary for onions to differ from beets, just as it's unnecessary for the world to exist at all. But the world does exist, upheld moment by moment by a loving God—not because it's necessary but because it delights Him. As His image bearers, our task is to see the world as He does: as something completely unnecessary and yet infinitely precious.

When we see food through this lens, delight becomes the natural response. And delight, as theologian Norman Wirzba suggests, is the key to gratitude. By cultivating delight, we learn to recognize and embrace the value of creation, entering a state of wonder that naturally leads to joy—and ultimately, thanksgiving. Wirzba writes, "Our thinking, if it is true at all, is maximally open to the wonder of the world, is properly amazed by it, and so slips, from time to time, into forms of praise."[84]

Any view of nutrition that strips eating of its proper delight—not in the sense of hedonistic indulgence, but in the innocent wonder and gratitude awakened by even simple, wholesome foods—is fundamentally flawed. Robert Farrar Capon goes further:

> "The world exists, not for what it means but for what it is ... Things, therefore, as things, are inseparable from God, as God. Separate the secular from the sacred, and the world becomes an idol shrouded in interpretations; creation becomes too meaningful to make love to."[85]

This assertion that food is inseparable from God may sound strange to some Christians, but it is profoundly biblical. Consider the Eucharist, where we partake of the "Bread of Life," whom John also describes as "the Word" made flesh. In modern English, "word" typically evokes a

---

84 Wirzba, *Food and Faith.*
85 Capon, *The Supper of the Lamb.*

simple unit of language made from letters, but for the Gospel's original audience, the Greek term *logos* carried a weightier meaning.

For ancient philosophers like Philo of Alexandria, the *logos* was the mediator between a holy, infinite God and a corrupt, finite world.[86] It was the divine logic or purpose that gave meaning to the physical world by embedding God's ideas in matter.[87]

By calling Jesus the *Logos*, John appealed to, but also revolutionized this idea: Jesus is not just a mediator or an abstract principle, but God Himself who enters into creation. He is the Creator, the logic behind all existence, and the redeemer of a world imprinted with His design. Creation, imprinted with this Logos, becomes a revelation of God's very self.

When we approach food from this perspective, eating becomes more than a mere necessity; it becomes an act of receiving God's self-offering love. Delight—and, by extension, gratitude—arises when we encounter food as a tangible reminder of God's perfectly created order and utterly unnecessary goodness.

Many of our diets, however, bear little or no trace of this divine Logos. Instead of reflecting the Creator's logic and love, much of what we eat, while consumable and tasting something like food, would be better described as "food-like substances." Picture Doritos, instant noodles, frozen pizzas, or sugary, fruit-flavored yogurts. Rather than bearing witness to the divine logic that transcends the material nature of food—inviting us to perceive it as a gift—such products embody the distorted logic of human ingenuity: a logic driven by instant gratification, extended shelf life, cheaper shipping, and cheaper labor.

By contrast, authentic food, which still bears the marks of its created purpose, nourishes both body and spirit. Here, taste precedes nutritional value, and flavor is no accident. It signals to our bodies about

---

86   Frédéric Louis Godet, *Commentary on the Gospel of John, with an Historical and Critical Introduction*, trans. Timothy Dwight, vol. 1 (New York: Funk & Wagnalls, 1886), 286–291.

87   Marvin R. Vincent, *Word Studies in the New Testament*, vol. 2 (New York: Charles Scribner's Sons, 1887), 25–33.

what we're about to eat and enables us to "taste and see that the Lord is good" (Ps. 34:8).

Food-like substances violate this sacred logic, deceiving our bodies with artificial signals while offering nothing to enrich our spirits.

Processed Foods

What do we mean by "processed foods"? Technically, even washing carrots is a form of processing, as are the many questionable steps required to make Cheese Whiz. Although the term generally has a negative connotation, it spans a wide range. At one end are wholesome practices like fermentation, cold pressing, stone grinding, and traditional curing, all of which preserve or enhance a food's natural qualities. At the other end are harmful methods—hydrogenation, bleaching, refining, artificial flavoring, and synthetic dyes—that strip nutrients and replace them with additives. While processing is not inherently problematic, *ultra-processing* is.

Studies estimate that more than half of the American diet is ultra-processed, a category that includes food-like substances made with ingredients not commonly found in home kitchens. These additives are designed to "imitate sensorial qualities of unprocessed or minimally processed foods and their culinary preparations or to disguise undesirable qualities of the final product."[88] In ultra-processed foods, such as most breakfast cereals, flavored yogurts, and lunch meats, flavor is divorced from real biological or spiritual value—and is often hostile to both.

How do we eat in a way that embodies gratitude and aligns with the Eucharistic paradigm—the ultimate model for theological eating? It begins with truly knowing and experiencing what we are grateful for. This requires recognizing the intrinsic value of food and embracing it as

---

88   Eurídice Martínez Steele, Dariush Mozaffarian, Joao B. Monteiro, Renata B. Louzada, and Carlos A. Monteiro. "Ultra-Processed Foods and Added Sugars in the US Diet: Evidence from a Nationally Representative Cross-Sectional Study." *BMJ Open* 6, no. 3 (2016): e009892.

an occasion for delight. Gratitude flows naturally when we perceive food not merely as a number or a collection of "good" and "bad" materials, but as a gift imbued with divine meaning.

This perspective deepens when we understand that Jesus's presence is not limited to the Lord's Supper. He is the *Logos*, the divine Word, who infuses every aspect of creation with His reason and love. He is both Sustainer and Participant in the world He made, and His perfect intent animates all of existence. When we see food as part of His work of creation—an expression of His very self—we realize that it is more than just sustenance. It is a living testimony to His self-offering love that calls us to respond with awe, delight, and sincere thanksgiving.

Thanksgiving doesn't just mean saying grace before a meal, though it certainly includes that. Rather, thanksgiving is the indispensable seasoning of every meal. It is the fundamental posture of a Christian, expressed even in the way we construct a diet that reminds us of the delightful experience God intends eating to be.

When Belief Becomes Biology

This may sound abstract and spiritual, but our perception of food can profoundly affect how our bodies respond to it. A 2011 study vividly illustrates this connection. Participants were given the same 340-calorie milkshake on two separate occasions but were led to believe differently about its nutritional content. On one occasion, they were told it was a modest 140-calorie "sensible" shake; on the other, they were told it was an indulgent 640-calorie treat.

The researchers measured how these perceptions impacted the participants' levels of ghrelin, a hormone that regulates hunger and satiety. Normally, ghrelin rises to stimulate appetite and falls to signal fullness after eating. The results were striking: After drinking the "sensible" shake, participants' ghrelin levels barely changed, leaving them just as hungry as before. In contrast, after drinking the "indulgent" shake, their ghrelin levels dropped significantly—by a factor of three— leading to a greater sense of fullness.

Remarkably, the participants' physical responses aligned with their expectations, not the actual nutritional content of the shake. This study underscores a profound truth: how we think about food can elicit tangible biological effects. A perception of indulgence can satisfy hunger, while a mindset of restriction can perpetuate hunger by keeping the appetite active. In essence, how we perceive food shapes how our bodies respond to it.[89]

Reconciliation

Would it come as a shock to learn that food does not simply materialize on supermarket shelves, ready to be "harvested" with the swipe of a card? For those accustomed to doorstep delivery, it can be equally startling to realize that online transactions do not magically conjure boxes of meat out of thin air.

In reality, food depends on countless others—on the interconnected workings of creation. As we have seen, relationship is woven into our fabric as bodies that are constantly both feeding on and feeding the rest of creation. Our physical need for sustenance points not only to our dependence on God, but also to the deeply relational core of our being, drawing us into the grand choreography of life.

Soil sets the stage, nurtures life, and cycles it through organisms small and large, ultimately ending up on our plates. When we become estranged from the complex network of bacteria, fungi, animals, and fellow humans who all contribute to this process, we also lose sight of the deeper value of food—a tangible reminder that our identity is most fully realized within a social fabric that extends beyond ourselves, and indeed beyond humanity.

Against this backdrop, Paul's sharp rebuke of the Corinthian Church for its unfaithful participation in the Lord's Supper remains

89   A. J. Crum, W. R. Corbin, K. D. Brownell, and P. Salovey, "Mind Over Milkshakes: Mindsets, Not Just Nutrients, Determine Ghrelin Response," *Health Psychology* 30, no. 4 (2011): 424–29.

relevant today. His warning against partaking of this sacrament in an "unworthy manner" speaks directly to our understanding of Eucharistic eating.

In his first letter to the Corinthians, he writes:

> "Whoever, therefore, eats the bread or drinks the cup of the Lord in an unworthy manner will be guilty concerning the body and blood of the Lord. Let a person examine himself, then, and so eat of the bread and drink of the cup. For anyone who eats and drinks without discerning the body eats and drinks judgment on himself." (1 Cor. 11:27–29)

Given the harsh consequences of guilt and divine judgment, it would be especially useful to understand what Paul meant by the phrase "unworthy manner."[90] The context suggests that Paul was disgusted with the unfaithful practices in Corinth that made a mockery of the Lord's Supper and amounted to an outright rejection of Christ's saving work. Research by New Testament scholar Richard B. Hays suggests that church members of higher social status were invited to more exclusive gatherings, where they dined and reclined on superior food and wine. Meanwhile, members of lower social status were left outside to partake of inferior offerings, creating a sharp divide within the early Christian community.[91]

By incorporating status distinctions recognized by pagan Roman culture into their practice of the Lord's Supper, the actions of the Corinthian Church violated the very nature of the event they were supposedly commemorating—one centered on unity in Christ, whose body and blood were sacrificed for the salvation of all who receive Him by faith, regardless of social status, race, and other arbitrary distinctions.

Paul then warns that failing to "discern the body" when partaking of the bread and wine is to "drink judgment" upon oneself. Over the

---

90   The original Greek phrase for "unworthy manner" in 1 Corinthians 11:27 is "ἀναξίως" (anaxiōs), which directly translates to "in an unworthy manner" or "unworthily."

91   Richard B. Hays, *First Corinthians* (Louisville: John Knox Press, 1997), 196, citing Pliny the Younger, *Letters* 2.6 (as cited in Schreiner and Crawford, *The Lord's Supper*, 79).

centuries, many Christians have understood this warning as a call to recognize the difference between the consecrated elements and ordinary bread and wine, or to acknowledge the significance of Christ's covenantal body represented in the meal. The ninth-century monk Ratramnus describes "discerning the body" as the "intelligent apprehension" of the Lord's body and blood, "perceived by the intuition of faith."[92] There is certainly merit to this interpretation, and it was likely at least part of what Paul had in view.

In context, however, Paul's repeated use of the word "body" to refer to the congregation of believers (as we explored in Chapter One) suggests that he is speaking primarily about the Church in this passage.[93] To "discern the body" in this sense is to recognize what it means to be united with Christ and to share in the sacred fellowship of His covenant people—a body in which all believers are members and gifts to one another.[94] Ratramnus elaborates on this aspect of the Eucharist:

> "It is also to be considered that in that bread, not only the body of Christ, but also the body of the faithful, is represented ... for it is made of many grains, even as the body of the faithful is increased by individual believers through the word of God. Wherefore as in a mystery that bread is taken to be the body of Christ, so also in a mystery are the faithful in Christ signified."[95]

By neglecting a Christ-centered fellowship in the Lord's Supper, the Corinthians were not truly sharing in Christ's death but were instead breaking the covenant and making themselves liable for His blood—identifying more with those who nailed Him to the cross than with His faithful followers.[96]

---

92 Ibid., 36.
93 Paul consistently uses this term throughout the letter to describe the collective body of believers unified in Christ (see 1 Cor. 10:16–17; 12:12–27).
94 Gordon D. Fee, *The First Epistle to the Corinthians*, rev. ed. (Grand Rapids, MI: Wm. B. Eerdmans Publishing, 2014), 564.
95 Ratramnus, *On the Body and Blood of the Lord*, 48.
96 Fee, *The First Epistle to the Corinthians*, 561.

Paul's instruction to avoid such guilt is therefore a call to sincere self-examination. This is not, as some have wrongly imagined, a demand to come to the table sinless or with more good deeds than bad tallied on the ledger—but rather an invitation to come rightly, with humility, repentance, and renewed joy in the assurance of forgiveness and new life in Christ. This call also reminds us that to partake worthily is to recognize not only the significance of Christ's sacrifice but also the covenant fellowship it establishes—affirming the unity of the Church as His body and the shared bond of grace that joins believers to one another.

The emphasis on covenantal unity echoes the Sermon on the Mount, where Jesus teaches:

> "So if you are offering your gift at the altar and there remember that your brother has something against you, leave your gift there before the altar and go. First be reconciled to your brother, and then come and offer your gift." (Matt. 5:23–24)

In other words, Jesus teaches that worship is empty unless we are first *reconciled* with our brothers and sisters.

If we are to eat *Eucharistically*, our ordinary diet should reflect this theme of reconciliation, but on an even broader scale.

Such eating involves receiving food as a means of communion—with God, with other people, and with the rest of creation. It should spur us to consciously assume "membership" in creation, a participatory role that reminds us that all of creation is upheld by the sustaining power of Christ, and which invites us to act as stewards rather than exploiters within this creation.

Practically, this means paying attention to how our food is produced, respecting the natural rhythms of the land, and acknowledging the broader consequences of our choices. Simply put, we must ask ourselves whether our food habits are fostering this sense of belonging in creation or reinforcing the estrangement that Jesus condemns in the Sermon on the Mount.

Contemporary, first-world societies have diets that are arguably more estranged than ever before. Most people are blissfully unaware of and largely disconnected from the origins of their food: the soil in which it was grown, the condition of the animals from which it came, the well-being of the farmer or rancher, and the extensive processing it underwent before appearing at the store or on the doorstep.

To illustrate this disconnect, consider the celebrated "successes" of the agricultural revolution. In the United States, we often praise the efficiency of a system in which only 1.3 percent of the population farms or ranches.[97] A former secretary of agriculture even boasted, "Because only one person in 43 is needed to produce food, others can become doctors."[98] Yet the tragic irony is that this "surplus" productivity is now struggling to address the very health problems created by our industrial food system. Even many American farmers no longer eat directly from their own soil—relying instead on frozen supermarket dinners.[99]

Farming and ranching were once called "husbandry," conveying a sense of marriage and mutual dwelling with the land. Genesis portrays husbandry as a dignified occupation that, until recently, occupied the time and affections of most of society and depended on the health and well-being of the soil, plants, and animals. This work not only fed people, but also sanctified them. Japanese farmer and philosopher Masanobu Fukuoka captured this sentiment when he said, "The ultimate goal of farming is not the growing of crops, but the cultivation and perfection of human beings."

In contrast, our modern system relies heavily on machinery, petrochemical fertilizers for depleted soils, and pesticides and herbicides to eradicate unwanted life. We have traded the labor of growing food for disconnected abundance—at the expense of our relationship to the land, its ecosystems, and the culture that food once nurtured.

Paul admonished the Corinthians for failing to discern the significance of the sacred meal as a tangible act of membership in the body of Christ. We make a similar mistake whenever we overlook the

---

97   USDA's NASS 2017 Census of Agriculture
98   Berry, *The Unsettling of America.*
99   Ibid.

sacramental nature of food as a sign and seal of our calling to be *members* of creation rather than mere consumers. When we eat according to God's design, however, we're less likely to make this mistake.

In Parts Two and Three of this book, we will explore how we can apply Paul's wisdom to our everyday food choices. We will focus on foods that enable us to participate fully and attentively in God's creation—foods that glorify the intricate web of life, respect the land and the people who tend it, provide for the animals that inhabit it, and ultimately nourish us as individuals made in God's image.

The Gift

A theology of food leads us to the inescapable conclusion that our deepest hunger is for Jesus, the only food that truly satisfies. The sacred meal—the Lord's Supper—is the most visceral and profound manifestation of this truth. In a sense, it epitomizes what food is intended to be: a tangible, nourishing revelation of God's self-offering love, through which He sustains us both physically and spiritually. How foolishly incongruous it is to profess this understanding when it comes to the Lord's Supper, only to otherwise subsist largely on food-like-substances that disconnect us from the reality that creation is a gift meant to draw us closer to our Creator! While we shouldn't diminish the Lord's Supper by trying to replicate its sanctity in everyday meals, we should at least seek opportunities for its meaning and effects to spill over into our daily eating—drawing closer to God in the way we source, prepare, and share food.

One of the most powerful insights of the Eucharist, evident in Jesus's words of institution—"given for you"—is the truth that His body and blood are presented as a total gift of self. This concept was explored earlier, noting how the body uniquely enables the person to express this reality. As we look at our own lives, we might ask: What kind of gifts are we? Are we offering gifts that are whole and life-giving, or ones that are diminished and unhealthy? How do our diets and lifestyles contribute to the quality of this offering?

In Jesus, we see the perfect embodiment of what it means to be fully alive, the Divine Physician who brings us into true health. Thus, as we seek a paradigm for nutrition that reflects our faith, we cannot stop at an understanding of Jesus as merely the Redeemed Body or the Bread of Life; we must also see Him as the perfect revelation of health—a theme that will guide the next chapter.

4

The Divine Physician
(A Theology of Health)

*"The blessing of life is a divine loan unmerited
by man ... Will he recognize and appreciate
the value of the gift? Will he realize that it
is given him in order that he may use, enjoy
and make it fruitful? ... Will he handle it as a
treasure which does not even belong to him,
of which he can dispose only according to the
purpose of the One from whom he has it, and
therefore not thoughtlessly nor arbitrarily,
but remembering that he must finally give
an account of his stewardship and use?"*

– KARL BARTH, CHURCH DOGMATICS

E ven more than eating and drinking, Jesus was known for healing.
The Gospels are filled with stories of Jesus's miraculous healings,
earning Him the nickname, "Divine Physician." He restored
physical well-being to the sick and offered spiritual liberation to the
possessed. He opened the eyes of the blind and the ears of the deaf,
inviting them to see and hear Him first, and He raised the dead as a
demonstration of His sovereign power.

Jesus's public healing demonstrations were often accompanied by the phrase, "Your faith has made you well," a theme that points to the profound meaning behind the miracles (Lk. 8:48, 17:19; Mk. 5:34). Some proponents of the so-called "health and wealth" gospel interpret this theme as a guarantee that faith in Jesus will bring health and prosperity in this life, placing it in the supremely oxymoronic category of Christian "self-help."

But despite Jesus's abundant compassion for the suffering people of his day, that's not the best lesson to draw from the multitudes of people who were made whole by their faith in His healing touch. Rather, we should see these acts as a foretaste of the much greater, eternal promise of health and wholeness that comes through faith in His redemptive work.

While perfect well-being, characterized by a seamless unity of body and spirit, eludes us in this earthly existence, God nevertheless desires a measure of health in our temporal lives. Not only must we come to terms with what this concept means from a Christian perspective, but we must also understand our role in promoting it, finding that this pursuit is ultimately a God-honoring form of stewardship with lasting—even eternal—significance.

Defining Health

Health is a term that means many things to many people.

The World Health Organization (WHO), taking somewhat of a holistic approach, defines it as "not merely the absence of disease or infirmity," but as "a state of complete physical, mental and social well-being."[100] Critics, however, rightly argue that this definition is far too broad: by including almost every aspect of personal well-being, it risks making health a catch-all category. There are a host of social factors, such as financial status, education, housing, and job satisfaction, that are only tangentially related to health but that this definition brings squarely within its purview. Distinguishing between health-related

---

100 "Constitution of the World Health Organization." World Health Organization. Accessed September 4, 2024. https://www.who.int/about/governance/constitution.

issues and broader societal challenges becomes difficult under this conceptualization.

At best, the WHO's "theory of everything" definition of health ends up meaning nothing. At worst, it places undue responsibility on healthcare professionals to address moral and social controversies—such as gender reassignment, abortion, and assisted suicide—that extend well beyond their medical expertise.[101] If our definition of health justifies practices that Jesus—were He a contemporary physician—would undoubtedly question, perhaps we should reconsider it.

In response to the WHO's expansive definition, some have called for a strictly scientific, value-free approach. Philosopher Christopher Boorse, for example, takes the opposite of the WHO's approach, defining health simply as "the absence of disease." But this seemingly straightforward definition inevitably raises an important question: what exactly is disease? To address this, Boorse describes disease as a condition that interferes with an organism's "natural function."[102] The problem with this definition, however, is that determining what is "natural" for a species—especially for the human species—is far from trivial or value-free.

One might say that a "healthy" heart can pump blood in a way that keeps a person alive and well. But who says that living is a natural function? From a Christian perspective, Thomas Aquinas's conception of the Natural Law suggests that preserving life is a duty, on the grounds that we can't be obedient to God if we aren't alive in the first place. The Sixth Commandment, in which God specifically forbids murder, also implies a broad respect for the preservation of human life. Neither line of reasoning, however, is purely scientific; both rely on moral and theological foundations.

Boorse's inclusion of reproduction as a "natural function" could also be challenged. While the biological process may be straightforward, various cultural and philosophical perspectives place different levels of

---

101   Neil Messer, "Toward a Theological Understanding of Health and Disease," *Journal of the Society of Christian Ethics* 31, no. 1 (2011): 163.

102   Christopher Boorse, "Health as a Theoretical Concept," *Philosophy of Science* 44, no. 4 (December 1977): 542–73.

importance on it. In contrast, Scripture regards marriage and procreation as complementary elements of God's plan, which involves propagating humanity throughout the earth.

These examples demonstrate that defining "natural functions"— and thus defining health—depends on a worldview that assigns meaning and purpose to human life. Therefore, despite his best intentions, Boorse's definition cannot remain purely value-neutral or scientific; value judgments inevitably creep in.

Therefore, having examined the pitfalls of worldly attempts to define health, we can now explore what health is according to this Christian perspective.

Swiss theologian Karl Barth may have captured it best, describing health as "strength for human life," a gift from God directed toward fulfilling our proper human purposes. [103] Christ is integral to this definition, for He embodies the flawless revelation of what it means to be human in the first place. As theologian and ethicist Neil Messer puts it,

> "We should not imagine that we can discover our proper ends, goods, or goals independently of God's self-disclosure in Christ, or that we can arbitrarily choose whatever goods or goals we happen to wish to pursue. Our goods and goals are given in Creation, and disclosed in and through Christ."[104]

Unlike Boorse's attempt to define health as a purely scientific concept, Barth's view unapologetically stems from a Christian worldview that recognizes humanity's nature and responsibilities before the Creator.

But unlike the WHO's sweeping definition, Barth avoids equating every dimension of well-being with "health," keeping it as a limited concept within a well-ordered context. Barth offers two specific clarifications that distinguish a Christian understanding of health from competing paradigms.

---

103 Barth, *Church Dogmatics*, 356.

104 Neil Messer. "Toward a Theological Understanding of Health and Disease." *Journal of the Society of Christian Ethics* 31, no. 1 (2011): 167.

A Good Among Goods

First, Barth emphasizes that health should be regarded as a "good among goods"—something of considerable worth, yet not an ultimate end. Like all gifts, health has inherent limits that are ultimately determined by God's sovereign will, the true source of all goods. The degree to which health should be prioritized varies according to the unique balance of goods before each person at any given time.

Martyrdom, for example, is a calling that many Christians have embraced, illustrating how the pursuit of health may give way to a higher purpose in service of God's will. Consider Stephen, who boldly preached before the Sanhedrin, an act that led to his stoning but also helped extend the gospel beyond Jerusalem. The same principle applies in less extreme circumstances, such as missionary work or charitable service in areas plagued by conflict, poor sanitation, and endemic diseases like malaria. Those who go abroad and accept these conditions in obedience to the Great Commission are not carelessly disregarding health; rather, they are prioritizing a greater good.

This comparative perspective does not lessen our responsibility to respect our lives and strive for the best possible health; it merely sets that pursuit in its proper context.

John Paul II echoed this sentiment in a 2005 letter on respect for human life:

> "Health is not, of course, an absolute good ... Properly understood, health nevertheless continues to be one of the most important goods for which we all have a precise responsibility, to the point that it can be sacrificed only in order to attain superior goods, as is sometimes demanded in the service of God, one's family, one's neighbor and the whole of society."[105]

---

105 John Paul II, *Letter to the President of the Pontifical Academy for Life and to Participants in the "Quality of Life and Ethics of Health" Congress*, February 19, 2005.

While affirming health as a good, he cautions that it is not absolute. Were it otherwise, health would sometimes clash with nobler ends that might be demanded in obedience to God's will.

An Enabler of Other Goods

Furthermore, health is neither an objective nor an intrinsic good; its value lies in supporting the legitimate purposes of human life as revealed by Christ. The goodness of vitality and strength consists in enabling the pursuit of our true human ends, but those ends, not health itself, hold ultimate meaning.

Imagine the emptiness of being "healthy" if it were disconnected from the essence of being human and living a fully realized life. A person who lives solely for health—obsessively pursuing remedies, supplements, and gadgets or retreating from society in search of pristine water and air—risks transforming health into an idol rather than recognizing it as a gift meant to serve higher purposes.

The biblical argument for the goodness of health hinges on its role as an enabler of greater goods. Health is not an end in itself but rather the means through which other noble ends become attainable. Through our bodies, we can strive to be gifts to our spouses, families, communities, and above all, living offerings to God. We are called to illumine the world with our works, serving as instruments of His will. Herein lies the true meaning of health.

In short, when health is understood as "strength for life," we transcend both worldly utopian ideals and purposeless indifference, placing health where it belongs—as one valuable good among others, directed toward the authentic purposes of human life.

An Eternal Perspective on Health

Now that we've defined health in a Christian context, it's important to develop a framework for why it matters. In other words, why is strength for life worth pursuing?

Karl Barth traces this mandate back to a biblical respect for human life. Because we are called to respect life in general, we should certainly respect our own lives, treating them as loans held in trust. If we are to give God any sort of return on this investment, we must obey His call to live fully human lives directed toward His purposes as revealed by Jesus. This entails a commitment to "will to be healthy," not as an end in itself, but as a means of gaining strength for our mission.

In other words, when we cultivate genuine health through disciplined habits, we prepare ourselves to bear fruit in service to God's purposes—fruit that will ultimately be rewarded with eternal gifts.

This idea can be controversial among Christians, but it need not be. We can rely solely upon *Christ's* finished work for our salvation—our works have no ability to justify and are thus meaningless in this regard. Yet Scripture repeatedly stresses the importance of our works. Jesus taught, "Whoever believes in me will also do the works that I do" (Jn. 14:12). Paul later emphasizes this sentiment in Ephesians, describing Christians as God's workmanship, "created in Christ Jesus for good works" (Eph. 2:10).

Though we might be tempted to separate our earthly from our eternal lives, Scripture presents the two as inherently intertwined. God insists our good deeds are "not in vain" and that Jesus will return "to repay each one for what he has done" (1 Cor. 15:58; Rev. 22:12). In other words, believers will receive rewards at Christ's judgment seat, where our sins are pardoned but our works are assessed.

According to Paul, "For we must all appear before the judgment seat of Christ, so that each one may receive what is due for what he has done in the body, whether good or evil" (2 Cor. 5:10). Paul vividly illustrates how our works—whether "gold, silver, costly stones, wood, hay, or straw"—will be tested by fire: the enduring ones will remain, while the worthless ones will burn up, sparing the individual but leaving him or her without treasure (1 Cor. 3:12–15).

This is the central point of the Parable of the Talents (Matt. 25). In this classic illustration of God-honoring stewardship, a master entrusts his wealth to servants and later evaluates the return on his investments. Two of the servants double their allotments—one servant turning five talents into ten, and the other turning two into four—and are equally congratulated when the master says, "Well done, good and faithful servant. You have been faithful over a little; I will set you over much" (Matt. 25:21). But the servant who buries his one talent without profit is condemned as a "wicked and slothful servant," and his single talent is given to the servant who was more fruitful. The master declares, "For to everyone who has will more be given, and he will have an abundance. But from the one who has not, even what he has will be taken away" (Matt. 25:19).

In this parable, Jesus emphasizes stewardship in terms of money, making it relatable and concrete. Many Christians readily apply this financial concept to tithing—offering a tenth part, or the "first fruits," of their labor. Yet, many of these same Christians, feeling good about their financial stewardship, neglect to steward their health, subsisting largely on Hot Pockets and Coke without thinking twice. Therefore, just as Jesus did, we might consider applying financial concepts to our management of health.

Using this analogy, Christian health author Scott Stoll introduces the idea of a "health bank account," where each healthy choice is like a deposit and each unhealthy choice a withdrawal. Steady, small "deposits" accumulate over time, fending off disease, maintaining vitality, and supporting a life that fulfills God's calling. The opposite occurs when the account is overdrawn—this is where the concept ceases to be a metaphor and takes a toll on our actual finances.

Injury and illness are leading causes of financial ruin, whether through crushing medical expenses or lost productivity. These consequences ripple outward, affecting family members who sacrifice their own time and energy to care for loved ones, taxpayers who shoulder the mounting costs of public healthcare and disability payments, health care workers whose talents could be applied elsewhere, and underserved communities that miss out on the outreach of healthy, vibrant volunteers.

Some may criticize the pursuit of health as a self-centered act, but seen in this light, neglecting health appears far more selfish. Balancing the "health bank account" is not just a personal duty but a service to others.

Aligning Identity and Action

James Clear, in his groundbreaking book *Atomic Habits*, argues that hopes and good intentions alone rarely produce lasting change. Instead, our habits flow from the identities we embrace.

For Christians, identity rests on the truth that we are members of the body of Christ, created for good works. Yet each person's role in that body is unique. Forming meaningful habits requires discerning which part of the body we are and what unique works we are called to accomplish.

- As citizens, we might seek better health to ease burdens on the social safety nets or to buck the flawed incentives of our healthcare system.

- As parents, we might prioritize an example of godly strength and abundance for our children, providing them with the energy they need from us.

- As sons and daughters, we might do the same for our aging parents.

- As church leaders, we might pursue health to effectively shepherd our congregations.

- As missionaries, health can help us stay in the field longer.

- As workers of all kinds, better health can extend our productive years, enabling us to continue serving, earning, and giving generously.

By integrating our sense of identity with our actions, we align our habits with our God-given roles, transforming the pursuit of health into an act of service and a reflection of divine purpose.

This concept of stewardship also sheds light on the moral dimension of health. Is it sinful to neglect one's health? How about making generally healthy choices, but indulging in the occasional bowl of ice cream or a soda? The writer of Hebrews helps answer these questions:

"Therefore, since we are surrounded by so great a cloud of witnesses, let us also lay aside every weight, and sin which clings so closely, and let us run with endurance the race that is set before us." (Heb. 12:1)

Life is framed here as an endurance race with an ultimate prize. But it's the difference between "weight" and "sin" that is particularly relevant in this verse.

By "lay aside every weight," the author is referring to a common practice of Roman athletes shedding weight—unnecessary gear, clothing, or perhaps even body weight—before a race. These "weights" aren't necessarily bad in themselves and may even be a blessing in the right circumstances but are things that for some reason or another could turn into an impediment.

This contrasts with a sin, which, by its very nature, is always a transgression of God's law and is allowable under no circumstances. While a weight might be a weight to one person and not a weight to the other, sins are always sins. Just like weights, the author encourages us to rid ourselves of sin like a runner would avoid traps and entanglements, lest he be snared during the race.[106]

Yes, certain sins—like gluttony or sloth—will inevitably sabotage health. But many unhealthy choices are better viewed as weights rather than sins: our unhealthy choices, especially when they become habits,

---

106 This distinction is reminiscent of the apostle Paul's sentiment, "'All things are lawful,' but not all things are helpful" (1 Cor. 10:23).

are like roadblocks that pile up and impede our ability to live according to God's purposes. This framework allows us to avoid applying strict legalism to health-related choices while still affirming their importance as a form of obedience to God's will.

Borrowing again from sound financial advice, a practical rule of thumb for health decisions is the 80/20 rule: the healthiest 80 percent of our choices determine how we handle the other 20 percent. In other words, if most of our actions are consciously health-affirming, then we've likely built a solid enough foundation to handle a few lapses in judgment, willpower, or knowledge that cause us to conform to the world's unhealthful ways. In doing so, we will likely still be amassing compound interest in our health bank accounts, or perhaps paying off some high-interest debt, all while keeping the eternal perspective in mind as the animating force behind our actions.

Ultimately, the Christian theme of stewardship is what animates a well-ordered will to be healthy. While God controls both our lifespan and health span, He entrusts much of their care to us. Fulfilling that trust allows us to live the abundant life He envisions, bearing fruit in this world and receiving rewards in the next.

Does Christianity Celebrate Weakness?

We've spent a great deal of time exploring the reasons to strive for strength, yet the Christian faith also reveals a shocking paradox: weakness can be a conduit of *God's* strength, and suffering can be an occasion for joy. As Paul says, "We rejoice in our sufferings, knowing that suffering produces endurance, and endurance produces character, and character produces hope" (Rom. 5:3–4).

But this doesn't mean that weakness or suffering is a virtue in itself; we should not actively seek them, nor should we invite them through careless choices. While God can redeem even our worst missteps, that does not grant us freedom to stumble recklessly. Rather, these moments of hardship remind us that when we reach the end of our own strength,

God's power can be made perfect in us, and authentic hope can take root.

What Does a Will to Be Healthy Look Like?

Finally, armed with a uniquely Christian definition of health—rooted in an embodied life in which our will to be healthy finds eternal meaning—we should naturally ask: What does this will look like? How do we begin improving our health?

Establishing a Baseline: The First Step Toward Stewardship

First, it is important to acknowledge that each person's capacity for health varies, shaped by a wide range of challenges. Many suffer from illnesses or injuries beyond their control—developmental disorders, genetic conditions, accidents, or harm caused by others. Such hardships can serve as catalysts for drawing closer to God, deepening faith, and fostering compassion. Others, however, experience conditions directly influenced by personal choices, such as poor lifestyle habits or unrepented sin.[107]

Regardless of the cause, gaining an honest understanding of one's current state of health is essential for meaningful improvement. This process begins with routine diagnostic testing, which provides a clearer picture of existing conditions and helps identify areas in need of change. The Appendix includes a comprehensive diagnostic plan for assessing key biomarkers, many of which are introduced in Part Two of this book, offering a practical framework for beginning to steward health in accordance with God's design.

Taking this initial step and making it a habit allows for greater clarity, intentionality, and faithfulness in the ongoing pursuit of strength for life.

---

107 Hebrews 12:5-7, 11; Revelation 3:19; John 15:2

Affirming a Mindset of Agency

A genuine commitment to health also requires the right mindset. Although often overlooked, this element of wellness is essential. The well-documented placebo effect demonstrates that belief alone can significantly influence the body's capacity to heal and remain strong. Everyone knows someone who is always talking about how sick they are—and, more often than not, they are. This is no coincidence. Chronic anxiety about illness or perceived illness can heighten stress, lower immunity, and even manifest physical symptoms that reinforce the fear.

Though God is sovereign over every outcome, this in no way diminishes the meaningful consequences of human choices. The first and most foundational of these—at least as far as health is concerned—is the choice to adopt a mindset of agency. A mind consumed by regret over past health decisions, lament over present conditions, or fear of what may come can be just as debilitating as any illness. By contrast, a mind oriented toward gratitude, purpose, and resilience can play a vital role in supporting healing and sustaining vitality.

A proper will to be healthy, therefore, is founded upon two key convictions:

1. "My present state of health, whatever it may be, is sufficient to accomplish God's purposes for me today."

2. "I have the capacity to meaningfully improve my health by making good choices."

By embracing both present strength and the potential for growth, it becomes possible to shift from a mindset of limitation to one of humble empowerment. This perspective fosters resilience, sharpens the ability to confront obstacles, and strengthens long-term commitment—making the pursuit of health not only attainable but sustainable. Ultimately, a disposition rooted in agency and hope provides the foundation for fully engaging in the pursuit of strength for life.

Embrace Stewardship: Owning the Inputs That Shape Health

With a clear understanding of one's current health status and a right view of personal agency under God's sovereignty the next step is to embrace the role of steward over the daily inputs that shape strength for life. Health, whether flourishing or failing, is experienced by the whole person, and it is not something delivered by institutions, but rather cultivated through faithful stewardship and intentional action. This integrative view stands in sharp contrast to the fragmented model of modern medicine.

Many people place the burden for their own health upon the "healthcare" system. But modern Western medicine, for all its notable achievements in emergency and acute care, is designed only to identify and manage disease through a "divide and conquer" approach. Under this model, issues such as fatigue, obesity, arthritis, anxiety, depression, and infertility are treated as isolated conditions, while chronic diseases such as cancer, Alzheimer's, and heart disease are assumed to be inevitable byproducts of aging. Many people see numerous specialists, each working in isolation to prescribe medications that manage a specific symptom, often exacerbating the other ones. This siloed, reductionist perspective treats patients not as wholes, but as collections of symptoms.

For this reason, healthcare often resembles a game of whack-a-mole with chronic disease. Most well-meaning doctors—overworked, constrained by ten-minute visits, and armed only with a prescription pad or scalpel—are ill-equipped to promote true health. But this shortcoming is nothing new. Consider the ailing woman in Mark's Gospel who "had suffered much under many physicians, and had spent all that she had, and was no better but rather grew worse" (Mk. 5:25–34). Only upon fighting the crowds to simply touch the threads of the Divine Physician's garment did she find healing from her debilitating hemorrhage. Today, as then, people spend fortunes—often subsidized by others—seeking help from a system that isn't set up to address root causes.

According to this healthcare—or "sick care"—model, "preventative medicine" is seen as a niche field. Holistic approaches, often the subject of mockery, are relegated to the category of "alternative medicine." But if we are to seek different health outcomes for ourselves and our families, we must begin to look at health care through a different lens. God's designs have always stood apart from prevailing norms. Why should our pursuit of health be any different?

A more holistic model, anchored in a reverence and awe of God's creation, recognizes each cell as a microcosm of the whole person. Our cells reflect the physical, mental, and, to some extent, even the spiritual aspects of our condition. When functioning effectively, they foster harmony across every dimension of health. This intricate design is no accident—it reflects a Creator who intricately weaves together every aspect of our being.

We have ample evidence that God desires our flourishing; after all, a single human cell contains a more potent healing potential than centuries of scientific effort combined.[108] By nourishing our cells as God designed—giving them what they need and withholding what they don't—we unleash this inherent power.

In this paradigm, willing to be healthy means gaining the knowledge and adopting the habits that let our cells, and thus our whole selves, flourish.

Three simple inputs determine our cellular health: building blocks, energy, and information. For example, stress management and mindfulness practices provide information to the cells in the form of signaling molecules that regulate hundreds of metabolic pathways in response to how we perceive ourselves or our environment. Exercise provides other messages, prompting cells to become more resilient and increase energy capacity. Sunlight, a less emphasized but critically important determinant of health, provides two of these key inputs: When received by photoreceptors in the eyes it acts as information, regulating circadian rhythms and orchestrating numerous physiological

---

108   Ben Rall, holistic health practitioner and the author of *Designed to Heal* (2023), popularized this insight.

changes. At the same time, sunlight serves as an energy input to convert cholesterol derivatives in the skin into vitamin D.

These and other lifestyle factors are critical determinants of health, but diet is certainly the most important factor under our control.

For decades, major corporations and respected public health institutions have promoted the damaging myth that "a calorie is a calorie," urging us to focus less on diet and more on exercise, as if food were simply a source of energy that exists in a balance. But while 100 calories of cookies and 100 calories of broccoli are the same according to the laws of thermodynamics, they have profoundly different effects on our cells. In truth, food is more than fuel—it also provides essential building blocks and, perhaps most importantly, it delivers information that guides how our bodies function.

The fatty acids and sugars we consume are the primary cellular energy substrates, releasing the sun's energy from double carbon bonds and harnessing it to produce the biological currency that enables all energetic reactions in the body. The amino acids we consume are the body's primary building blocks, becoming the structural proteins, enzymes, neurotransmitters, antibodies, and other materials that make life possible. Our cells, and therefore our bodies, are literally printed from these materials, starting in the womb and continuing every day until we die. Finally, micronutrients from food provide the cell with information about the world around it by regulating gene expression, acting as cofactors in various enzymatic reactions, and influencing a litany of cellular processes.

As flawed as the prevailing healthcare system may be, it is often a symptom of a deeper issue: a poor diet. As outlined in the Introduction, societal factors play a significant role in fueling dietary confusion. We demonize traditional foods like whole, raw milk as threats, yet deem highly processed grains—grown with fossil-fuel fertilizers, soaked in herbicides, and dyed with artificial colors—a viable part of a "balanced" diet.

Still, none of this removes personal responsibility. Despite these challenges, individuals retain the agency to make wise choices—to overcome confusion through discernment, and to reshape habits in ways that align with truth. Health is not ultimately dictated by institutions or trends, but by the daily decisions that reflect one's stewardship of the body entrusted by God.

This theological understanding of the body, food, and health forms the foundation for a distinctly Christian approach to nutrition. It reveres our bodies as masterpieces of God's handiwork, embraces food as a tangible expression of His self-giving love, and recognizes health not as a substitute for the gospel but as a foretaste of a superior heavenly reality to come. God calls us to promote and protect this gift of health as a tool for living fully human and fruitful lives as we persevere toward this reality—the first and perhaps most important step is to repair our broken relationship with food.

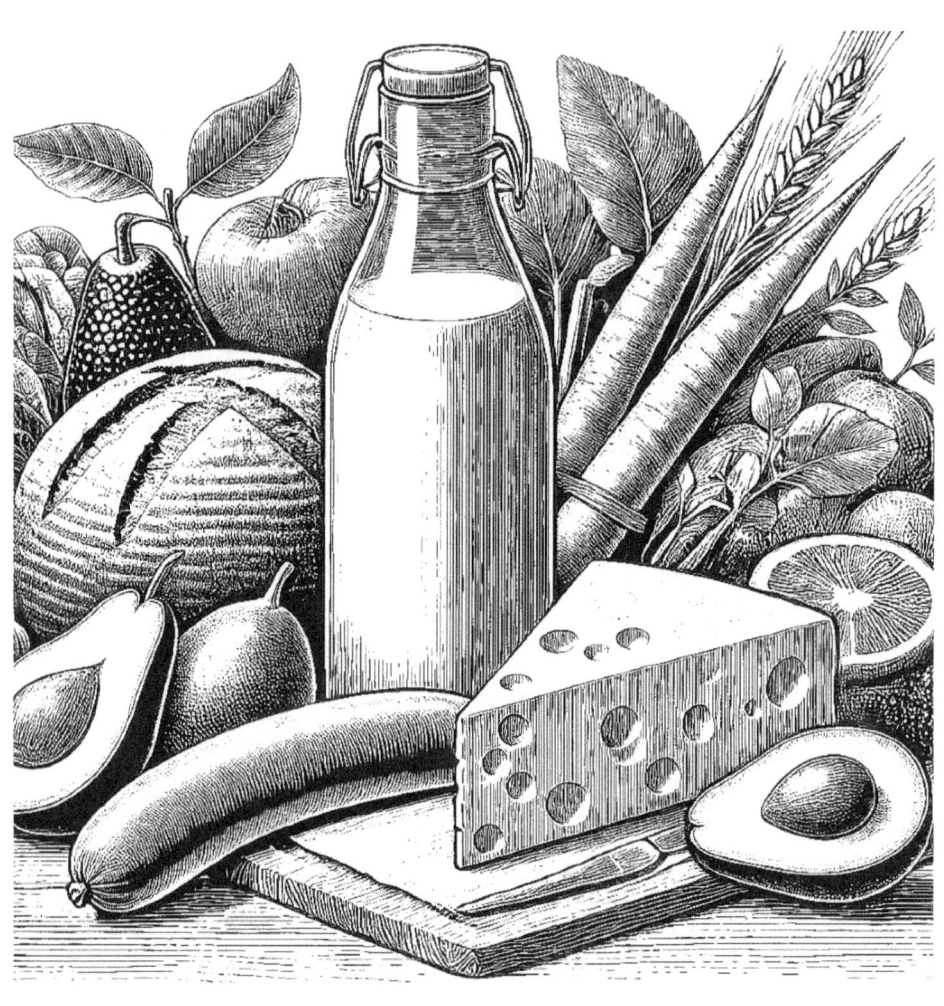

PART II

God's Design for Nutrition

*"People are fed by a food industry which pays no
attention to health,
and are treated by a health industry
which pays no attention to food."*

– WENDELL BERRY

E quipped with a theological perspective on nutrition—a perspective that places the body, food, and health in a larger spiritual context—we now face a practical question: how do we proceed?

This question is unique to our modern era because, until relatively recently, most people had few choices when it came to food. For countless generations, the human experience revolved around the struggle to put *any* food on the table, a task that required the combined time, effort, and resources of nearly everyone in a community. Availability depended on natural factors such as season, soil quality, climate, and limited trade. As a result, people ate mostly what was grown or raised nearby, relying on simple preservation methods like salting, fermenting, or drying. All of this food was "real" and "minimally processed"— though such terms did not require definition—and gratitude came more naturally, given both the considerable effort required to produce it and the very real alternative of not having it at all. In many ways, this made the "Eucharistic" approach to eating—one marked by gratitude, reconciliation, and discernment—far more intuitive than it is today.

After generations of free trade and global markets, modern societies now enjoy what economist Julian Simon calls "superabundance," a level of productivity that generates a massive surplus of resources at minimal cost.[109] Where people once worried about *whether* they would eat, we now largely struggle to decide *what* to eat and how not to *overeat*. This is both good and bad.

In 1900, the leading cause of death was infection, a problem that medical science has nearly eradicated. Today, however, five of the seven leading causes of death—heart disease, cancer, cerebrovascular disease, Alzheimer's disease, and diabetes[110]—are, as Part Two will show, either directly caused by or inextricably linked to metabolic dysfunction, once virtually nonexistent.

---

109 Gabe L. Pooley et al., "The Simon Abundance Index: A New Way to Measure Availability of Resources," *CATO Policy Analysis* no. 857, December 2018.

110 David S. Jones et al., "The Burden of Disease and the Changing Task of Medicine," *New England Journal of Medicine* 366, no. 25 (June 2012): 2333–38.

When it comes to food, superabundance means options and convenience, but also less connection to the objective world that created it, fewer obvious reasons for delight, and more potential stumbling blocks. But while we have more choices in how we make and fuel ourselves, the fundamental laws of health remain the same, making it all the more important for us to understand and align ourselves with them.

Chapter Five examines key aspects of the body's metabolism—the set of cellular processes that handle energy, building materials, and information derived from food. Although the human body is irreducibly complex and not fully understood from a scientific perspective, a basic grasp of its metabolic systems is sufficient to guide meaningful change.

Chapter Six argues that most, if not all, chronic diseases are symptoms of a broader, underlying issue: metabolic dysfunction—the cellular inability to mobilize sufficient energy while eliminating waste. This unifying root is gaining increasing attention in scientific research. To better understand this multifaceted disease in more digestible terms, it's important to become familiar with its sign, its key drivers, and its common underlying contributors.

Finally, with a clear picture of metabolic dysfunction, we turn to how diet can help or hinder our cells. Specifically, Chapter Seven explores what *not* to eat, while Chapter Eight focuses on what *to* eat. Rather than offering a simple list of "good" versus "bad" foods, we'll explore a set of dietary priorities aimed at supporting the body's most essential metabolic processes. Though these aren't the only considerations, they form a practical foundation for dietary habits that we'll refine in Part Three.

5

Fearfully Made (Embracing God's Design in Human Physiology)

"And men go abroad to admire the
heights of mountains, the mighty billows
of the sea, the broad tides of rivers, the
compass of the ocean, and the circuits of
the stars, and pass themselves by;"

– AUGUSTINE, THE CONFESSIONS OF SAINT
AUGUSTINE, BOOK X, CHAPTER VIII

The holistic model of health approaches the body as if it were fearfully and wonderfully made by a purposeful Creator. Seeking to understand creation—especially our own bodies—has therefore always been understood as a small glimpse into the mind of God, or what philosopher of science Stephen Meyer calls, "a secondary source of authoritative revelation about the character and wisdom of the Creator."[111]

Echoing this sentiment, the sixteenth-century reformer John Calvin observes,

---

111   Stephen C. Meyer, *The God Hypothesis: Three Scientific Discoveries That Reveal the Mind Behind the Universe* (New York: HarperOne, 2021), 41.

"Our wisdom, insofar as it ought to be deemed true and solid wisdom, consists almost entirely of two parts: the knowledge of God and of ourselves. But as these are connected together by many ties, it is not easy to determine which of the two precedes and gives birth to the other."[112]

As we seek to uncover and embrace God's design for nutrition, let's begin by examining our own design, focusing on metabolism. While it's enormously complex, we can at least gain a basic understanding by identifying its key components and understanding how they work together. Through this lens, we'll begin to explore how God's fearful and wonderful design allows us to manage the information, building blocks, and energy we receive from food.

The Gut (the Front Line of the Metabolism)

Of all the body's metabolic systems, the gut—the "front line" of the metabolism—is the focal point. As the receiver and initial processor of food and our most direct connection to the world around us, it's as though our bodies are literally constructed around this focal point.

Leon Kass vividly captures the centrality of the gut:

"Topologically and digestively speaking, the bodies of higher animals are, in fact, highly complex variations of a simple plan: a thick-walled solid cylinder built around a hollow tube that runs through its center. In schematic cross-section, the organism is like a doughnut, nourished from its hole, here and there armed with appendages that work either to keep that hole filled or to keep the doughnut from filling some other doughnut's hole."[113]

What Kass humorously calls the "doughnut hole" is at the root of both health and disease. The ancient Greek physician Hippocrates

---

112 John Calvin, *The Institutes of the Christian Religion*, I.I.1, trans. Ford Lewis Battles (Philadelphia: Westminster Press, 1960).

113 Kass, *The Hungry Soul*, 23.

recognized this truth nearly 2,500 years ago when he said, "All disease begins in the gut." Indeed, it seems that Hippocrates was *way* ahead of his time, as modern science continues to uncover the profound implications of gut health for overall well-being.

At its most basic level, the gut converts ingested food and drink into absorbable nutrients—carbohydrates, fats, proteins, vitamins, and minerals—which pass through the intestinal walls into the bloodstream to nourish tissues and organs throughout the body. But while this basic process has been understood for centuries, we've only recently begun to appreciate the extent to which it is facilitated by trillions of microbial helpers, collectively known as the gut microbiome.

As mentioned in Chapter One, this diverse community of microbes inhabiting the gastrointestinal tract plays a critical role in determining how food is processed and utilized. Much like fingerprints, each person's microbiome is unique—like a "metabolic fingerprint." But unlike fingerprints, these microbial profiles have tangible significance for our quality of life.

The influence of the gut microbiome is evident in how specific microbial profiles correlate with specific health outcomes. For example, studies show that germ-free mice develop high blood pressure when they receive fecal transplants from humans with hypertension.[114] Similarly, an "obesity microbiome," characterized by lower levels of Bacteroidetes, higher levels of Firmicutes, and generally reduced bacterial diversity, is often observed in obese individuals.[115] Even neurological conditions like Autism Spectrum Disorder (ASD) have been linked to gut imbalances, with some cases showing improvement or complete reversal when healthy gut compositions are restored through probiotics or fecal

---

114 Jing Li et al., "Gut Microbiota Dysbiosis Contributes to the Development of Hypertension," *Microbiome* 5, no. 1 (February 2017) (as cited in Steven R. Gundry, *Gut Check* [New York: HarperCollins, 2024]).

115 Chika Kasai et al., "Comparison of the Gut Microbiota Composition Between Obese and Non-obese Individuals in a Japanese Population, as Analyzed by Terminal Restriction Fragment Length Polymorphism and Next-generation Sequencing," *BMC Gastroenterology* 15, no. 1 (August 2015) (as cited in Gundry, *Gut Check*).

transplants.[116] One of the most amazing (and alarming) statistics demonstrating the overall impact of the gut on health is that the use of antibiotics in childhood leads to a 44 percent increase in the likelihood of developing mental health issues later in life.[117]

But how could this simple hollow tube have such a profound effect on the rest of the body, influencing diseases seemingly far removed from digestion?

The answer lies in the gut's role as the body's first point of contact with food. The gut doesn't just distribute nutrients; it also relays critical information about the outside world, preparing the body for challenges and offering protection from invaders. This complex interplay is optimized by fostering a diverse and resilient microbial ecosystem.

Although they don't have ears to hear or a mouth to speak, gut microbes are highly effective communicators. They produce metabolites—a fancy word for bacterial poop—that serve as signals, nutrients, or chemical messengers in the gut. These metabolites enable cooperation among microbial species, each performing specialized tasks such as aiding digestion or signaling the immune system.

Amazingly, these cooperative systems are enhanced by a process called "quorum sensing," whereby bacteria collectively decide on actions once they detect sufficient levels of metabolites to confirm that their population has reached a productive threshold, known as a quorum.

However, these microbes are not always cooperative. While some populations cooperate, others compete, making the ecosystem more resilient. This competition fosters a healthy balance, as rival microbial populations drive each other to become more robust, contributing to the overall stability of the gut microbiome.

The metabolites produced by a diverse and resilient gut microbiome provide numerous benefits throughout the body. For example, when

---

116 Zuzanna Lewandowska-Pietruszka et al., "Microbiota in Autism Spectrum Disorder: A Systematic Review," *International Journal of Molecular Sciences* 24, no. 23 (November 23, 2023): 16660.

117 Katherine Dinan and Timothy Dinan, "Antibiotics and Mental Health: The Good, the Bad and the Ugly," *Journal of Internal Medicine* 292, no. 6 (July 12, 2022): 858–69, https://doi.org/10.1111/joim.13543.

microbes ferment soluble fiber, they produce short-chain fatty acids (SCFAs) like acetate, butyrate, and propionate. These SCFAs act as signaling molecules that influence various cellular processes throughout the body. Butyrate, in particular, supports colon health, strengthens the gut barrier, reduces inflammation, and supports energy balance.

Taken together, these discoveries, while only a mere appetizer compared to what modern research has uncovered, suggest that the gut is more than a site of digestion—it is a dynamic command center for metabolic regulation, immune signaling, and whole-body health. As we become more aware of our interconnectedness with the rest of creation—that we are both a host and are hosted in numerous ways— we not only learn more about the logic of God's designs, but hopefully gain an appreciation for cultivating these relationships and reaping the benefits for our health.

DNA, Epigenetics, and Building Blocks

King David suggested that we are "knitted together" by the hand of God (Ps. 139:13–14). Thousands of years later, our understanding of the double-helix structure of DNA—which zips and unzips to create the proteins that make up our bodies—makes this knitting analogy feel less like a metaphor and more like a scientific reality.

As we've seen, the human body is dual in nature: physical material animated by a distinct and enduring form. In these terms, we can understand our dietary material as being trans-*formed* into more of us according to an invisible yet very real in-*form*-ation. At the cellular level, this phenomenon occurs through the interplay of our genetic material, building blocks (particularly amino acids), and chemical signals from outside the cell.

For a long time, we only vaguely understood this process, considering DNA to be a static blueprint that deterministically dictates traits by directing the assembly of proteins in a manner akin to an architect's plans. This perspective fostered the belief that the genetic codes for health, obesity, cancer, and even certain behaviors were hardwired from conception. Only recently have we discovered that an additional layer of information from the outside—largely from the food we eat—regulates the "expression" of these genes, determining when they are activated or silenced. This understanding redefines DNA as less of a blueprint and more of a menu of potential options that respond to environmental inputs.

The example of female honeybees illustrates how identical DNA can lead to vastly different developmental outcomes based on environmental factors, specifically diet.

Within the matriarchal framework of the colony, workers and queens occupy distinct roles and exhibit pronounced differences in organs and body structures, to the extent that they hardly resemble the same species. Workers, who vastly outnumber the queens, are infertile and equipped with stingers and pollen baskets. In contrast, queens are significantly larger, fertile, lack both a stinger and pollen baskets, and live much longer lives. Remarkably, despite these divergences, all female bees start out as clones with identical DNA, challenging the simplistic notion that genes alone dictate their outcomes.

The striking differences in their development are entirely due to their diet. But it's not just the quantity or quality of food that accounts for these significant differences. Rather, it's how the food interacts with the bees' DNA. Initially fed a special baby formula known as royal jelly, most female bees eventually switch to a different "worker diet." The lucky few who are chosen to be queens, however, feed exclusively on royal jelly their entire lives. This royal diet triggers hormonal changes that activate the "queen" genes while silencing the "worker" genes, resulting in the dramatic differences between the two.[118]

Royal jelly, as it turns out, is quite good for humans, too. But while eating it, or anything else for that matter, won't change humans in such striking ways, the same basic mechanisms apply to us and profoundly influence our health.

---

118 David S. Moore, *The Developing Genome: An Introduction to Behavioral Epigenetics* (New York: Oxford University Press, 2015).

Many nutrients act as signals to the cell, turning specific genes on or off. Vitamin D, for example, binds to a receptor that interacts with DNA to activate genes that produce antimicrobial peptides, thereby bolstering the immune system.

Lifestyle factors can also influence *long-term* gene expression patterns without altering the underlying DNA sequence. A well-documented example of this phenomenon is that of the Dutch Hunger Winter, a period of famine during World War II. Pregnant women who experienced severe malnutrition during this period had children who, decades later, had altered gene expression related to their early exposure to nutrient deprivation. The affected genes were related to growth and metabolism, so these survivors had higher rates of obesity, diabetes, and cardiovascular disease later in life.

The processes that determine how genes are turned on and off are called "epigenetic"—meaning "above" or "beyond" the genes—because they occur at the interface between the DNA and its environment. As a result, the signals our environment sends to our DNA have as much influence on cellular programming as the genetic code itself.

While the DNA we inherit at birth remains unchanged, it is constantly shaped by the epigenome—a dynamic layer of molecules that adapts to environmental cues over time. These molecules do not alter the underlying DNA sequence, but instead regulate which parts of the genome are expressed by either promoting or blocking their transcription into proteins. Beginning in the womb (and perhaps even before conception) the epigenome helps our cells adapt to their environment, either promoting health or susceptibility to disease.[119]

This ability of the epigenome to respond to environmental signals, including diet, once again underscores the important role of food as more than just a source of energy and building blocks, but as critical information that helps the body align itself with external rhythms and conditions. The long-standing debate about the roles of nature

---

119 The epigenome can act as a family history, as some lifestyle habits are transmitted to offspring. In the case of the Dutch Hunger Winter, the epigenetic effects were detected several generations later. But the extent to which the epigenetic code is inherited is still a topic of scientific inquiry.

versus nurture is increasingly clarified by our understanding that the information presented to our cells is just as vital as the genetic blueprint itself. The epigenome not only responds to lifestyle and environmental inputs, but also stores this data in a kind of "metabolic memory" that guides our cells.

Our DNA is therefore not a static set of instructions, but a responsive player that adjusts our key metabolic processes based on external influences, with massive implications for our overall health.

Energy Production and Regulation

While we've now begun to explore how our bodies manage the information and building blocks we consume, we haven't delved into what most people associate with food: the energy it provides.

While calories aren't everything, understanding how the body manages energy is essential. Many of our metabolic processes are dedicated to regulating energy intake, storage, and expenditure, and disruptions in this system can lead to disease.

Therefore, we'll discuss the three key players in this system: our mitochondria, our energy management organs, and our energy management hormones.

Mitochondria

Mitochondria are the organelles inside almost every cell in the body that high school biology textbooks refer to as the "powerhouses of the cell." They earn this title because one of their critical tasks is to convert adenosine diphosphate (ADP), much like an uncharged biological battery, into adenosine triphosphate (ATP), the fully "charged" version that powers almost all cellular processes.[120]

Before mitochondria revolutionized energy production, ancient cells relied solely on glycolysis, a process that breaks down glucose

---

120 The cell uses this energy currency by snapping off the third phosphate group, which converts the ATP back to ADP.

into pyruvate and generates just two molecules of ATP per glucose molecule. Glycolysis is quick and doesn't require oxygen, making it ideal for anaerobic conditions, such as moments of intense exercise when the lungs can't keep up with demand. Even today, some cells depend entirely on glycolysis. For example, red blood cells, which lack mitochondria altogether, exclusively use this process to meet their energy needs. Cancer cells, too—largely cut off from the body's oxygen supply due to rapid, disorganized growth—rely on glycolysis to fuel their growth.

In contrast, cells with mitochondria can achieve vastly greater energy yields. Mitochondria process pyruvate (from the breakdown of glucose in glycolysis)—and other fuel sources like fatty acids and ketones—through aerobic respiration, generating approximately 15 times as much ATP per molecule of glucose than glycolysis alone. This efficiency makes mitochondria indispensable for fueling the body's energy-intensive processes.

Mitochondria's ability to utilize multiple types of fuel makes them highly versatile energy producers. They convert these diverse raw materials into a universal fuel molecule, acetyl-CoA, which enters the Krebs (or citric acid) cycle. This cycle generates high-energy electrons, which are then harnessed in a process called the electron transport chain (ETC) to complete the yield of roughly 30 molecules of ATP.

This is where oxygen comes in to make advanced life on earth possible. Oxygen molecules, with two unpaired electrons in their outer orbitals, are highly reactive and eager to accept additional electrons. Acting like a powerful electromagnet, oxygen drives the flow of high-energy electrons generated by the Krebs cycle through a series of protein complexes embedded in the mitochondrial membrane. At the end of the chain, oxygen combines with hydrogen to form water. But this water is a mere byproduct; the real magic happens in the flow of electrons through the ETC, which essentially generates electrical energy.

This electrical energy powers ATP synthase, a turbine-like enzyme that spins at an astounding 96,000 revolutions per minute. The mechanical energy from this motion enables the enzyme to attach extra phosphate groups to ADP molecules, converting them into ATP—the charged energy currency that powers nearly every function in the cell.

It's an elegant and highly efficient system, a testament to the intricate design of our Creator.

But while mitochondria are best known for producing energy, their role extends far beyond powering cells. Responsible also for epigenetic and hormone regulation, among a host of other tasks, they are increasingly recognized as the master regulators of the cell.

Epigenetic Regulation. Mitochondria influence gene expression by sending signaling molecules to the nucleus, integrating the cell's metabolic state with genetic regulation. This communication determines which genes are activated or silenced, profoundly affecting cellular behavior. Morley Robbins, a prominent researcher and founder of the Root Cause Protocol, suggests that while our genes are controlled by epigenetics, our epigenetics are ultimately controlled by mitochondrial energetics.[121]

Hormone Regulation. Mitochondria are also indispensable for hormone regulation. Not only do they provide the ATP needed for hormone synthesis, but they also house key enzymes required for the production of hormones such as cortisol, estrogen, and testosterone. For example, the conversion of cholesterol to pregnenolone, the precursor for all steroid hormones, occurs exclusively in mitochondria, underscoring their central role in hormone biosynthesis.

This remarkable versatility and centrality to cellular function are further reflected in how mitochondria are distributed and maintained within different types of cells, tailored to meet the varying energy demands of the human body.

Roughly 1,500 genes in human DNA are considered "mitochondrial genes," encoding the proteins needed to maintain mitochondrial function. However, mitochondria also have their own genetic material, which allows them to maintain a degree of independence. This autonomy includes the ability to divide and replicate as needed to meet the energy demands of the cell.

---

121 Morley Robbins, *Cu-RE Your Fatigue: The Root Cause and How to Fix It on Your Own* (Columbus, OH: Gatekeeper Press, 2021).

Cells with higher energy requirements, like those in the heart and liver, contain significantly more mitochondria—heart cells can have about 10,000 mitochondria each, while liver cells contain about 2,000. In contrast, most other cells tend to have on the order of 100 mitochondria per cell.

In summary, healthy and robust populations of mitochondria are essential for cellular function. Their adaptability, capacity for efficient aerobic respiration, and regulation of genetic and hormonal processes make them indispensable for managing metabolic energy and maintaining overall health. Far from being merely the cell's "powerhouses," mitochondria act as master regulators, orchestrating the intricate symphony of life at the cellular level.

Key Energy Management Organ Systems

Understanding mitochondria helps us grasp how cells generate energy, but to fully appreciate energy distribution on a larger scale, we must examine how specialized cells within the body's energy management systems function uniquely to regulate and allocate energy.

To introduce another financial analogy, the bloodstream functions as the body's metabolic "wallet," holding a small, readily available supply of energy "cash" for immediate use. But just as most people wouldn't carry their entire life savings on their person in the form of cash, the bloodstream isn't designed to hold excessive amounts of energy.

This raises a key question: how does the body maintain *just enough* readily available cash in the metabolic wallet to meet cellular demands without accumulating toxic levels in the bloodstream? The answer lies in the coordinated efforts of three critical organ systems—the liver, adipose tissue, and skeletal muscle—each fulfilling a unique role in managing the body's energy balance.

The Liver. A powerhouse of energy management, the liver manages, converts, and stores energy in various forms to maintain a steady supply for the body. In our financial analogy, it functions as a metabolic cashier, financial broker, and checking account—a true metabolic Swiss Army knife, essential in both times of famine and abundance.

After a meal, when there's an influx of "cash" into the bloodstream, the liver switches to "deposit mode." It removes excess glucose from the blood and converts it into glycogen—a compact, rapidly accessible form of stored energy—through a process called glycogenesis. Glycogen is stored primarily in the liver and muscles, providing a readily available reserve for maintaining blood sugar levels during fasting or physical activity. However, the liver's capacity to store glycogen is limited to about 100–120 grams (approximately 400–500 calories). Once glycogen stores are full, the liver converts the excess glucose into triglycerides (fat) through de novo lipogenesis, a metabolic process that transforms carbohydrates into fatty acids. Some triglycerides remain stored in the liver itself, but the majority are packaged into lipoproteins and sent into the bloodstream for long-term storage in fat cells. In addition to managing glucose, the liver also processes fatty acids, which it can either use for its own energy needs or package and distribute to adipose tissue for storage.

When blood glucose levels drop, such as during fasting or after intense exercise, the liver goes into "withdrawal mode." It breaks down its stored glycogen into glucose through a process called glycogenolysis and releases it into the bloodstream to ensure that cells continue to receive energy even in the absence of dietary glucose. Once glycogen stores are depleted, the liver initiates gluconeogenesis, a metabolic pathway that synthesizes glucose from non-carbohydrate sources like amino acids (derived from muscle protein), lactate (produced by muscles during anaerobic activity), and glycerol (from fat breakdown). This dual ability to release stored glucose and create new glucose enables the liver to sustain energy levels during prolonged fasting or periods of high demand.

In short, in its capacity as "cashier," the liver is constantly at work managing the body's energy "cash flow," regulating the intake, storage, and release of energy substrates based on the body's needs. As a "financial broker," it converts energy between different forms—glucose, glycogen, and triglycerides. As a "checking account," it even stores a small and accessible reserve of these currencies (particularly glycogen) for times of greater demand.

Adipose Tissue. While the liver serves as a short-term energy buffer, adipose tissue acts as the body's "savings account," storing substantial energy reserves for extended periods of time—enough that one morbidly obese individual famously fasted for over a year, surviving only on his body fat.[122]

Far from being an inert blob, body fat is a dynamic organ that plays a role in regulating appetite, immune function, and other physiological processes, all while serving as a reservoir of excess energy.

Fat cells, or adipocytes, function like balloons, capable of expanding up to 1,000 times their original size to store triglycerides. These adipocytes cluster into three primary types of fat tissue, each with distinct effects on health:

1. Subcutaneous Fat: The most abundant type, subcutaneous fat is the flabby stuff that is distributed throughout the body and located just under the skin. While primarily responsible for storing excess energy, it also insulates the body, cushions muscles and bones, and serves as a conduit for nerves and blood vessels.

2. Visceral Fat. Unlike subcutaneous fat, visceral fat accumulates only within the torso. Nestled under the abdominal muscles, it competes for space among vital organs such as the liver, pancreas, heart, and intestines. While subcutaneous fat is metabolically benign, visceral fat is inherently inflammatory and contributes to the development of disease. In recent years, a new classification has emerged in medical literature to describe individuals who appear thin but carry substantial amounts of visceral fat in their torso: "Thin on the Outside,

---

122 Angus Barbieri, once weighing 465 pounds, undertook a medically supervised extended fast in 1965 that lasted 382 days. He survived on only water, tea, coffee, and vitamin supplements during this time, reducing his weight to 180 pounds by the end of the fast.

Fat on the Inside" (TOFI). This condition is increasingly recognized as a serious health risk.

3. Ectopic Fat: The most harmful form (even more so than visceral fat), ectopic fat accumulates in ideally non-fatty organs, such as the liver (i.e., fatty liver disease) or muscle, where it disrupts organ function and promotes inflammation. While marbling in a ribeye may be desirable, "marbling" of human organs is far from ideal.

Deposits into adipose tissue come from two main sources: circulating glucose and triglycerides. Both forms of energy are converted into lipid droplets for long-term storage in fat cells through processes like lipogenesis and de novo lipogenesis. Withdrawal later occurs via lipolysis, the process by which fat is broken down into free fatty acids and glycerol and then released into the bloodstream to fuel muscles, the liver, and other tissues. In a healthy metabolism, this withdrawal process is seamless, allowing the body to efficiently mobilize fat for energy during fasting, exercise, or low-carbohydrate diets. In an unhealthy one, accessing stored fat can become a challenge, like trying to withdraw gold bars from a locked vault.

Skeletal Muscle. While many people recognize muscle for its role in movement and strength, fewer realize that skeletal muscle is also a metabolic organ—and a highly intelligent one, at that. Skeletal muscle is increasingly being recognized as perhaps the body's most important metabolic organ and, according to physician and muscle health expert Gabrielle Lyon, the "organ of longevity."[123]

As the largest organ in the body (for most people), skeletal muscle can store glucose as glycogen, much like the liver. But the true metabolic power of muscle lies in its ability to *use* this energy. Muscle tissue can fuel

---

123 This title reflects not only skeletal muscle's role in energy management but also its roles in preventing injuries in elderly people, serving as an amino acid reservoir for repair and recovery after injury or illness and releasing anti-inflammatory myokines during contraction, which contribute to immune system regulation and reduce chronic inflammation.

its own mitochondria with stored glycogen, or it can draw both glucose and fatty acids directly from the bloodstream to meet energy demands.

In our financial analogy, maintaining adequate muscle mass is like having access to a powerful "spending spree." During periods of high energy demand, muscle consumes a large portion of the body's energy reserves, ensuring that glucose and fatty acids are put to use.

But even at rest, muscle remains metabolically active. Unlike fat, which passively stores energy, muscle tissue requires a steady calorie input just to maintain itself. This elevated resting metabolic rate underscores the essential role of skeletal muscle in energy management and overall metabolic health.

Together, the liver, adipose tissue, and skeletal muscle form the cornerstone of the body's energy management system. The liver balances short-term energy availability, adipose tissue provides long-term reserves, and skeletal muscle ensures efficient energy utilization. These organs work in harmony to keep our mitochondria supplied with the substrates they need for energy production without overwhelming the bloodstream with toxic levels of glucose or fatty acids.

However, this coordination is not automatic. None of these organs instinctively knows when to store energy or when to release it. So how do they communicate and regulate these processes?

The missing piece is the body's intricate network of signaling molecules, especially hormones, that orchestrate these processes and maintain balance.

Key Energy Management Hormones

Hormones serve as the body's primary chemical messengers, enabling communication between organs and cells. Produced by glands throughout the body, hormones travel through the bloodstream to target cells equipped with specific receptors. When a hormone binds to its receptor, it conveys critical information about the body's internal or external environment, prompting cells to adjust processes such as gene expression, metabolism, and energy balance. The primary function of hormones is to maintain homeostasis—a fancy word that describes a state of balance and stability within the body's systems. Feedback mechanisms are essential to this process, ensuring that hormones are released when needed and cease production when their job is done.

While hormones perform a myriad of regulatory functions throughout the body, we'll focus on those that have an outsized impact on regulating our energy resources.

Thyroid Hormone. Thyroid hormone, produced by the thyroid gland, regulates heart rate, body temperature, and the rate at which the body burns calories. Acting as a "metabolic throttle," high levels of thyroid hormone speed up metabolism, while low levels slow it down. Imbalances can lead to weight gain, fatigue, or other metabolic issues.

Ghrelin and Leptin. In the realm of appetite regulation, ghrelin and leptin play opposing roles. Ghrelin, known as the "hunger hormone," is produced primarily in the stomach and signals the brain when it's time to eat, stimulating appetite and encouraging food intake. On the other hand, leptin, known as the "satiety hormone," is produced by fat cells and signals the brain that the body has sufficient energy stored, helping to suppress appetite and prevent overeating. Leptin plays a particularly crucial role in long-term energy balance, acting as the body's gauge of fat stores. Together, ghrelin and leptin perform a delicate balancing act, tightly regulating food intake and energy storage to meet the body's needs.

Insulin and Glucagon. The most critical hormones in energy regulation are insulin and glucagon, which work in complementary opposition to manage blood sugar levels and energy storage. Insulin is produced by the pancreas in response to rising blood glucose levels, typically after a meal, and has the primary function of lowering blood glucose by sending it to all cells that will take it. As an anabolic (growth) hormone, it facilitates the uptake of glucose into cells by binding to insulin receptors on cell membranes and opening the metabolic port of entry. Once inside, the glucose is either used for energy, stored as glycogen (in liver and muscle cells), or stored as fat (in the liver and adipose tissue).

On the flip side, glucagon, insulin's counterpart, is released by the pancreas when blood glucose levels drop, such as during fasting or strenuous exercise. Glucagon signals the liver to enter "withdrawal mode" and release glucose to buffer levels in the blood. Additionally, glucagon prompts fat cells to release fatty acids into the bloodstream, offering an alternative fuel source for the body when glucose availability is limited.

When all these hormones work in harmony, they maintain energy balance by regulating glucose levels, controlling fat storage and mobilization, and adjusting the metabolic rate based on the body's needs. This finely tuned hormonal system allows the body to respond dynamically to different conditions, ensuring that we have enough energy to meet our needs without overloading the bloodstream or starving the cells.

Fearfully and Healthfully Made

Given this brief exploration of our core metabolic processes, it is clear that our bodies are not only fearfully and wonderfully made, but they are intricately designed to promote health and vitality. Every system, from the gut to the mitochondria to the DNA, works together to harness God's sustaining power through food—to convert the light energy in its chemical bonds into ATP, to respond to the information it provides us from the outside world, and to build and repair our structural materials with its biological bricks.

Soon, we will explore what kind of food our bodies—particularly our guts, mitochondria, and DNA—expect us to eat. Conversely, we'll discover what kinds of food-like substances to avoid in order to promote strength for life.

But first, in the next chapter, we will build on this physiological introduction by considering not how it's *supposed* to work, but how it goes wrong. Contrary to popular belief, disease is not necessarily hardwired into our genes, nor is it willed by our Creator. Nevertheless, it remains a very real program that our cells switch to when they aren't given the right stuff. These consequences, stark and undeniable, offer perhaps the best insight into how we can prevent chronic illness through diet.

6

The Root of Disease (Understanding Metabolic Dysfunction)

> *"The realm of death which afflicts man in the*
> *form of sickness, although God has given it*
> *power and it serves as an instrument of His*
> *righteous judgment, is opposed to His good will*
> *as Creator ... To capitulate before it, to allow*
> *it to take its course, can never be obedience*
> *but only disobedience towards God ... A little*
> *resolution, will and action in face of that realm*
> *and therefore against sickness is better than a*
> *whole ocean of pretended Christian humility*
> *which is really perhaps the mistaken and*
> *perverted humility of the devil and demons."*
>
> – KARL BARTH, CHURCH DOGMATICS

Karl Barth, who described disease as the "messenger of death," offers a profound theological perspective on sickness. He saw it as a manifestation of humanity's fallen condition—an obstacle to life and health that stands in opposition to God's original intent. Disease is not good in itself nor part of God's creational blessing, but rather a consequence of the corruption introduced by sin. Yet even this suffering unfolds under the sovereignty of God's providence, who, though not responsible for sin or evil, ordains all things for His purposes—including judgment, discipline, and ultimately redemption. If health is strength for life, then disease can be understood as "weakness opposed to this strength."[124] It is a formidable adversary that we are commanded to resist, but we can only resist this enemy if we are familiar with it.

In this context, metabolic dysfunction emerges as the most prevalent modern form of this messenger of death. As we've explored, food—God's grace made delicious—is more than just energy. It also provides the information and building blocks necessary for cellular repair and maintenance. However, when the body fails to properly use these nutrients while managing the exhaust, cellular dysfunction ensues, and the consequences ripple throughout the entire system.

Metabolic dysfunction lies at the root of many of today's most common chronic diseases—conditions as diverse as chronic fatigue, heart disease, infertility, cancer, diabetes, and neurodegenerative disorders.

So, what exactly *is* metabolic dysfunction? Where does it come from? Answering these questions is the business of this chapter.

Unlike the traditional Western medical model, which often focuses on diagnosing and managing isolated symptoms, we'll explore the deeper, fundamental causes of disease. By understanding these underlying issues, we can better examine how our diets either contribute to or help prevent metabolic dysfunction.

This chapter will focus on:

1. Recognizing metabolic dysfunction, particularly through its hallmark sign—insulin resistance.

2. Exploring the two-headed monster that drives metabolic dysfunction: inflammation and oxidation.

3. Identifying key contributors to this dysfunction, including mitochondrial dysfunction, leaky gut, and mineral imbalances.

---

124 Barth, *Church Dogmatics*, 363.

By understanding these underlying causes, we'll lay the groundwork for the dietary principles discussed in the next chapters—principles designed to optimize our strength for life and resist any weakness opposed to this strength.

The Sign: Insulin Resistance

Metabolic syndrome, once known as "syndrome X," first gained widespread recognition as a medical condition in the 1980s. However, it wasn't until 1998 that the WHO established a formal definition that allowed for a clearer diagnosis. According to this definition, metabolic syndrome is identified by the presence of insulin resistance along with any two of the following: high blood pressure, dyslipidemia (i.e., low HDL cholesterol and/or high triglycerides), central obesity, or protein in the urine (a sign of kidney damage).

The emphasis on insulin resistance reflects its centrality to metabolic dysfunction and its role as the most reliable marker of the condition.

What is Insulin Resistance?

As discussed in the previous chapter, insulin is a hormone produced by the pancreas that regulates blood glucose levels. After a meal, insulin facilitates the uptake of glucose by tissues—primarily the liver, muscles, and fat cells—reducing blood sugar. Insulin also suppresses the liver's production of glucose and promotes the conversion of excess glucose into fat for storage.

Insulin resistance occurs when the body's cells become less responsive to insulin's signals, leading to elevated blood sugar levels despite high levels of circulating insulin. This resistance often begins in specific tissues, later becoming systemic.

Skeletal muscle is often the first major tissue to develop insulin resistance, reducing its ability to act as a glucose sink. As a result, the liver may also become resistant, failing to respond to insulin's storage signals and continuing to release glucose into the bloodstream unnecessarily. Meanwhile, adipose tissue often remains sensitive to insulin, absorbing excess glucose and converting it into fat. Only when insulin resistance affects multiple tissues is the entire body considered insulin resistant.

When insulin becomes less effective at signaling cells to absorb glucose, the pancreas compensates by producing more insulin to maintain normal blood glucose levels. This state of chronically elevated insulin, known as hyperinsulinemia, poses serious health risks, as we'll explore later. However, the real issue lies in how the brain interprets these metabolic signals: it mistakenly perceives low cellular energy availability despite high blood sugar levels. In response, the brain triggers appetite and raises the blood glucose setpoint, reinforcing the cycle.

Over time, this hormonal chaos creates a harmful feedback loop: blood glucose levels rise, the pancreas works overtime to produce insulin, and the body becomes increasingly resistant to its effects. The result is the paradoxical state common in modern society: being *overfed* yet *undernourished*. Excess energy is stored as fat, but the body struggles to access these reserves for fuel, leading to persistent fatigue, increased hunger, and further weight gain.[125]

A Flawed Understanding of Insulin Resistance

Despite its significance, insulin resistance is often overlooked in clinical practice. The medical establishment has well-known standards for type II diabetes and even "prediabetes," but it often fails to recognize that these diagnoses are just stops along the continuum of insulin resistance. This is because diabetes has long been viewed indirectly through the lens of glucose, not insulin.[126] In fact, insulin levels aren't even tested on a standard blood panel. Instead, physicians continue to diagnose prediabetes and diabetes by their respective fasting glucose thresholds,

---

125 This phenomenon occurs especially if adipose tissue still responds to insulin's storage signal.

126 This is partly because insulin has, until recently, been more difficult to measure, and also because diabetes was first diagnosed by a hallmark symptom—sweet urine—which greatly influenced the general association between diabetes and sugar.

both of which are reached long—often decades—after insulin resistance has set in.

The pancreas can compensate by producing excess insulin for years, masking the problem until its ability to keep up is exhausted. By the time fasting glucose levels rise, metabolic dysfunction is already well advanced.

Pre-diabetes?

The term "prediabetes" is profoundly misleading. When a patient's fasting blood glucose level reaches the 100–125 mg/DL range and the physician diagnoses prediabetes, it is commonly assumed that he or she is simply "at risk" of developing a disease. This couldn't be further from the truth. A prediabetic has already progressed significantly along the spectrum of insulin resistance and shows evidence of a deeply dysfunctional metabolism—a disease in itself.

Because insulin resistance is characterized by excess insulin in the blood, it could easily be diagnosed in its earliest stages by a simple fasting insulin blood test—even when fasting blood glucose levels are still in the "normal" range of 100 mg/DL or less. The HOMA-IR test is the gold standard for detecting insulin resistance and is simply calculated from fasting blood glucose and insulin levels, providing a measure of how efficiently the body uses insulin to control blood glucose.

$$\text{HOMA} - \text{IR} = \frac{\text{Fasting Insulin } \left(\frac{\mu U}{mL}\right) \text{ x Fasting Glucose } \left(\frac{mmol}{L}\right)}{22.5}$$

The higher the number, the greater the insulin resistance, with a number above 2.0–2.5 beginning to indicate an unhealthy condition.

The Consequences of Hyperinsulinemia

Chronically elevated insulin levels have widespread effects on the body, contributing to:

Cardiovascular Disease. Remember, insulin is primarily a growth hormone. Thus, one of its effects on the cardiovascular system is the excessive growth of smooth muscle cells in blood vessels, leading to narrowing of the arteries, inflammation, and plaque formation. It also damages the delicate lining of blood vessels (the endothelium), making them more susceptible to inflammation and plaque formation. Finally, chronically elevated insulin causes the kidneys to retain sodium, raising blood pressure—a major risk factor for heart disease.

Obesity. Hyperinsulinemia drives the storage of fat, especially visceral and ectopic fat, both of which are associated with metabolic complications.

Cancer. Again, as a growth hormone, insulin can promote the uncontrolled cell proliferation characteristic of cancer.

Worsening Insulin Resistance. As if heart disease, obesity, and cancer weren't enough (on top of the many other effects of hyperinsulinemia), elevated insulin levels worsen insulin resistance![127] It's similar to building a tolerance to caffeine: the more coffee a person drinks, the less noticeable its stimulating effects become.

But beyond being a stand-alone risk factor, insulin resistance acts as a flashing warning sign of a deeply disordered metabolism. When cells resist insulin's signals, they essentially "close the door" on glucose, signaling that they are unable to effectively process or store it. But why are insulin-resistant cells so resistant to this vital energy source?

To answer this question, we need to examine the key drivers of metabolic dysfunction that push cells to this breaking point: inflammation and oxidation.

---

127 Joseph A. M. J. L. Janssen, "Hyperinsulinemia and Its Pivotal Role in Aging, Obesity, Type 2 Diabetes, Cardiovascular Disease and Cancer." *International Journal of Molecular Sciences* 22, no. 15 (2021): 7797.

The Key Drivers: Inflammation and Oxidation

Inflammation and oxidation are distinct yet interrelated processes that play a central role in driving metabolic dysfunction, often manifesting as insulin resistance. To understand how these forces undermine metabolic health, let's first explore oxidation.

When we think of oxidation, oxygen naturally comes to mind. As previously discussed, the oxygen molecule's two unpaired electrons make it highly reactive, acting like an electromagnet—a property that our mitochondria utilize in the electron transport chain to produce ATP. But God's design for complex life relies on an element that can be just as toxic as it is vital, as this same reactivity can be destructive if left unchecked. Oxygen can steal electrons from or bond with other molecules, producing reactive oxygen species (ROS)—molecules that both result from and contribute to oxidation.

Most people understand oxidation as the catalyst for things like forest fires, explosions, and rusting metal, but few realize the extent to which it can also "rust" or "smolder" within our bodies. Oxidation in the body can damage critical cellular components, including lipids, proteins, and DNA, often setting off a chain reaction of damage that spreads throughout cells and tissues.

The body has a natural defense system against oxidation: antioxidants. These molecules freely donate electrons to neutralize ROS without destabilizing themselves, thereby combating oxidative stress. However, when ROS levels overwhelm the body's antioxidant defenses, oxidative stress ensues, damaging tissues and increasing the risk of chronic disease.

Inflammation, although related to oxidation, is a distinct phenomenon. While oxidative stress is simply an imbalance between ROS and antioxidants that tips the body into a reactive state, inflammation is a natural immune system response aimed at protecting and healing the body. Derived from the Latin *inflammare*, meaning "to burn," inflammation has rightly earned a bad reputation, but it is critical for responding to acute injuries such as wounds, infections, or sprains. Without this response, the body wouldn't be able to mitigate the assaults of everyday life on earth. It's only when inflammation occurs at the wrong time or in the wrong dose that it turns from a healing process into a destructive one. Chronic, widespread inflammation—akin to a smoldering fire—not only diverts precious energy from other necessary processes, but it also disrupts these critical metabolic processes and fuels metabolic dysfunction.

The connection between inflammation and a variety of disease states is well documented. For example, research shows that acute infections tend to make the body less sensitive to insulin by disrupting insulin signaling pathways.[128] Similarly, there is an intriguing link between periodontitis (gum disease) and type 2 diabetes. Given that both diseases are associated with sugar consumption, it's not hard to imagine why people with diabetes would be more likely to develop gum disease. But it may be a bit more surprising to learn that the reverse is also true; the inflammatory response to gum disease is known to cause insulin resistance.[129] Chronic inflammatory diseases such as rheumatoid arthritis, Crohn's disease, and lupus also exacerbate insulin resistance.[130, 131] Even obesity, often considered a passive condition, plays an active role in metabolic dysfunction. Overfilled fat cells release inflammatory molecules called cytokines that interfere with normal cellular functions, especially in muscle and liver tissue. These cytokines can convert ectopic fat into ceramides, a type of fat that directly disrupts insulin signaling.[132]

Modern medicine often treats these conditions—whether diabetes, gum disease, or obesity—as isolated events or genetic misfortunes.

128 E. C. Drobny et al., "Insulin Receptors in Acute Infection: A Study of Factors Conferring Insulin Resistance," *The Journal of Clinical Endocrinology and Metabolism* 58, no. 4 (1984): 710–16.

129 Brian Chee et al., "Periodontitis and Type II Diabetes: A Two-Way Relationship," *International Journal of Evidence-Based Healthcare* 11, no. 4 (2013): 317–29.

130 Cecilia P. Chung et al., "Inflammation-Associated Insulin Resistance: Differential Effects in Rheumatoid Arthritis and Systemic Lupus Erythematosus Define Potential Mechanisms," *Arthritis and Rheumatism* 58, no. 7 (2008): 2105–12.

131 Nicole Bregenzer et al., "Increased Insulin Resistance and Beta Cell Activity in Patients with Crohn's Disease," *Inflammatory Bowel Diseases* 12, no. 1 (2006): 53–56.

132 Benjamin T. Bikman and Scott A. Summers. "Ceramides as Modulators of Cellular and Whole-Body Metabolism," *Journal of Clinical Investigation* 121, no. 11 (2011): 4222–4230.

However, they are deeply interconnected and have a bidirectional relationship with metabolic dysfunction: they are caused by it and help exacerbate it, primarily through the process of inflammation.

This brings us back to oxidation, a major source of stress that triggers inflammation. When oxidative stress overwhelms the body, the immune system perceives it as an assault and triggers an inflammatory response. This creates a vicious cycle: oxidative stress fuels inflammation, which generates more ROS, exacerbating tissue damage and perpetuating insulin resistance.

Together, inflammation and oxidation form a destructive feedback loop at the heart of metabolic dysfunction. But they don't happen spontaneously. As we dig deeper into the roots of metabolic dysfunction, we must become familiar with three common causes of inflammation and oxidation: mitochondrial dysfunction, leaky gut, and key mineral imbalances. Understanding these causes will help us develop strategies to prevent or reverse the cycle of metabolic dysfunction and restore health and balance to the body.

Contributors to Inflammation and Oxidation

Mitochondrial Dysfunction

Recall from the last chapter that mitochondria are the master regulators of metabolism, orchestrating complex processes that yield clean and robust energy production. But their central role in cellular health also means that any disruption in their function naturally has far-reaching consequences. Metabolic dysfunction, as we'll see, is almost synonymous with mitochondrial dysfunction.

Ideally, mitochondria function much like a well-tuned car engine, producing clean "exhaust" in the form of water and carbon dioxide. But even the best engines produce some "smog." In the cell, this smog comes from ROS, which are formed in the mitochondria when electrons leak from the ETC and prematurely bind to oxygen instead of producing water and powering ATP production. In small amounts, these ROS aren't inherently harmful. They even serve a useful purpose, acting as signals that help cells adapt to stress by triggering antioxidant defenses. Problems arise, however, when ROS production outpaces the mitochondria's ability to neutralize them, which creates a state of oxidative stress.

This oxidative stress first damages the mitochondria themselves, undermining their ATP production. But its damage doesn't stop with the current generation of mitochondria. Mitochondrial DNA (mtDNA), which is housed within the mitochondria, is 16 times more susceptible to ROS damage than human DNA, which is shielded within the cell's nucleus. When mtDNA is damaged, it leads to faulty replication, creating a downward spiral of increasingly dysfunctional mitochondria, reduced energy output, and escalating oxidative stress.[133]

In essence, when mitochondria are overloaded or poisoned, they succumb to harmful levels of oxidative stress; when they are damaged, they intensify it. Cells overwhelmed by this stress try to protect themselves by rejecting excess fuel—this is why they stop responding to insulin's signal.

But the damage doesn't stop there. As Casey Means points out, mitochondrial dysfunction also triggers chronic, widespread inflammation. The body's immune cells, as mighty as they are, struggle in vain to assist an underpowered and ailing cell. They can't fix the real causes of this dysfunction—a bad diet, poor sleep, excessive stress, lack of movement, or insufficient sunlight—so they resort to their natural playbook: recruiting more immune cells and sending out more inflammatory signals.[134] This, of course, compounds the issue and creates a smoldering fire throughout the body.

Ultimately, impaired energy production in the mitochondria is the heart of metabolic dysfunction, as it promotes widespread inflammation and oxidation and leaves the body without the energy for essential

---

133   Kelsey H. Fisher-Wellman and P. Darrell Neufer, "Linking Mitochondrial Bioenergetics to Insulin Resistance via Redox Biology," *Trends in Endocrinology and Metabolism* 23, no. 3 (2012): 142–53.

134   Casey Means and Calley Means, *Good Energy: The Surprising Connection Between Metabolism and Limitless Health* (New York: Avery, 2024).

tasks—from muscle contraction to glucose regulation in the liver. As we'll see, diet is a major contributor to this phenomenon, but first there are a couple other significant contributors to oxidation and inflammation to explore.

Leaky Gut

Our "doughnut holes" are lined with a thin (only one cell thick) layer of epithelial cells supported by a protective layer of mucus. This lining serves as a selectively permeable barrier, allowing nutrients to enter the bloodstream while keeping harmful substances out. The integrity of this barrier is closely tied to the health and diversity of the gut microbiome— the trillions of bacteria that live in the digestive tract. When the microbiome is compromised or the gut barrier is weakened, the barrier can become permeable, allowing harmful substances to escape from the gut and enter the bloodstream. This condition, commonly referred to as "leaky gut," is not often formally diagnosed but can significantly contribute to widespread inflammation.

To illustrate this phenomenon, one particularly nasty class of particles known to cross a leaky gut barrier are lipopolysaccharides (LPS), fragments of bacterial cell walls. Colloquially known as "little pieces of sh*t," LPS wreak havoc once they enter the bloodstream, triggering systemic inflammation linked to conditions such as obesity, heart disease, rheumatoid arthritis, and other inflammatory disorders.[135]

But while LPS are one of the worst inflammatory agents known to invade a leaky gut, they aren't the only ones. Inflammatory plant proteins called lectins, pathogenic bacteria like E. coli, and even undigested food particles from otherwise healthy foods such as broccoli can provoke inflammatory responses. In people with food intolerances, the immune system reacts to these leaked particles by producing antibodies that lead to chronic inflammation whenever the offending food is consumed.

---

135   Martin J. Page et al., "The Role of Lipopolysaccharide-Induced Cell Signalling in Chronic Inflammation," *Chronic Stress* 6 (February 8, 2022): 24705470221076390.

Even more concerning is a phenomenon called molecular mimicry. Certain plant proteins that cross the gut barrier resemble human proteins. When the immune system encounters these look-alike proteins, it releases inflammatory cytokines with a mug shot of the offender, rallying immune cells to attack. With the immune system on high alert, it may attack anything that looks even remotely like the perpetrator, even if it's a human protein. For example, when thyroid proteins are mistaken for these offending plant proteins, the result can be Hashimoto's thyroiditis, an autoimmune disease that damages the thyroid. Other autoimmune conditions such as rheumatoid arthritis, psoriasis, and multiple sclerosis can also be traced back to the same process of inflammation driven by a leaky gut.[136]

A healthy gut—and by extension, a strong gut barrier—not only prevents inflammation caused by leakage but also helps reduce oxidative stress by supporting mitochondrial health. As previously mentioned, the gut microbiome produces SCFAs, such as butyrate, which confer several systemic benefits. Among these key benefits is butyrate's ability to protect mitochondria by promoting a process called mitochondrial uncoupling.

During uncoupling, mitochondria temporarily stop producing ATP and generate heat instead, essentially "wasting" energy. While this may seem inefficient, it serves a vital purpose: relieving mitochondria of the oxidative byproducts ("smog") produced during ATP synthesis, allowing them to rest and recover. Moreover, this process stimulates the production of new mitochondria, improving the cell's ability to meet future energy demands without generating excessive oxidative stress. In effect, mitochondrial uncoupling acts as a powerful antioxidant mechanism, reducing oxidation at its source.

In summary, when the front line of the metabolism fails, systemic inflammation is the inevitable result.

A leaky gut allows harmful substances to infiltrate the bloodstream, fueling chronic inflammation and increasing the risk of autoimmune and metabolic disorders. Conversely, a healthy gut not only prevents

---

136 Gundry, *Gut Check*.

inflammation, but also supports mitochondrial function, reduces oxidative stress, and protects the body from metabolic dysfunction.

Mineral Dysregulation

A third, and lesser-known contributor to the oxidation and inflammation that underlies metabolic dysfunction is mineral dysregulation, specifically imbalances in three essential metals: iron, magnesium, and copper.

It may come as a surprise that iron can be a major contributor to oxidative stress in the body. After all, iron, of all metals, is a symbol of strength and vitality, so much so that foods with added iron are said to be "fortified," as if they make the body more robust. And while iron is indeed necessary for the production of red blood cells and the transport of oxygen throughout the body, it has a dark side when present in excess.

As mineral researcher Morley Robbins notes, "Iron is, without question, the metal that ages us … Iron is the master pro-oxidant element on planet Earth and is the principal element behind what is called oxidative stress."[137]

This paradox of iron's duality became clearer in the early 1980s when pathologist Jerome Sullivan proposed the "Iron Hypothesis."

Sullivan sought to explain several puzzling trends in heart disease: Why does the risk of heart disease increase with age, and why do women enjoy relative protection during their menstrual years but catch up with men after menopause? Moreover, why is the disease virtually nonexistent in impoverished and malnourished societies? While these trends were largely dismissed as "facts of life," Sullivan saw a unifying factor: iron accumulation.

The Iron Hypothesis essentially posits that heart disease risk correlates with the body's iron load. Women lose iron through menstruation, and malnourished people consume and store less iron,

---

137 Robbins, *Cu-RE Your Fatigue.*

both of which reduce oxidative stress-related damage.[138] But how is this possible when so many people are told the opposite—that they are low in iron and should supplement their intake with pills?

Iron's potential toxicity in the body stems from the fact that it doesn't mix well with oxygen. Like a rusty car exposed to the elements, excess iron in the body is prone to oxidation. One particularly damaging reaction involves hydrogen peroxide (H_2O_2), a type of "smog" produced by the mitochondria's ETC. Through the "Fenton reaction," iron donates an electron to H_2O_2, converting it to the hydroxyl radical (OH), the most reactive and damaging form of ROS. These radicals wreak havoc on cells and tissues, promoting inflammation and oxidative damage.

Despite being discovered back in 1894, the implications of the Fenton reaction remain underappreciated. But it's simply a fact that unbound iron tends to accumulate in the body's most metabolically active organs, such as the heart and liver, making these organs particularly vulnerable to oxidative stress. This may explain why iron overload is linked to diseases like heart disease, liver disease, and metabolic dysfunction.[139]

This phenomenon challenges the widely held belief that cholesterol is the primary culprit in heart disease. Instead, Sullivan argues that cholesterol is an anti-inflammatory compound, an innocent bystander that occasionally gets caught up in the oxidation caused by excess iron. "The iron hypothesis redefines the cholesterol hypothesis," he notes. "Cholesterol and lipoproteins become, not culprits, but victims, targets of iron-catalyzed reactions."[140]

Eugene Weinberg, an iron expert, argues that humans are designed to live in a delicate balance between iron deficiency and iron

---

138   Jerome L. Sullivan, "Iron versus Cholesterol—Perspectives on the Iron and Heart Disease Debate," *Journal of Clinical Epidemiology* 49, no. 12 (December 1996): 1345–52.

139   Lisa A. McDowell, Pujitha Kudaravalli, Richard J. Chen, and Kristin L. Sticco, "Iron Overload," in StatPearls, updated June 5, 2023, accessed January 24, 2025, https://www.ncbi.nlm.nih.gov/books/NBK526131/.

140   Ibid.

sufficiency.[141] His research emphasizes that while iron is essential for life—playing key roles in hemoglobin formation, mitochondrial energy production, and thyroid hormone synthesis—excessive iron stores are harmful, accumulating in tissues and contributing to oxidative stress. Weinberg critiques the common misconception that "more is always better" when it comes to nutrition, suggesting that while iron serves a necessary purpose in the body, excess stores can be detrimental.

Enter magnesium, a mineral now recognized as critical to overall health, yet chronically deficient in most people. It is well known that over 300 enzyme reactions throughout the body require magnesium, but even that may be an understatement, as one study found magnesium binding sites on a whopping 3,751 human proteins.[142]

Most notably, magnesium is indispensable for energy production, particularly in processes like glycolysis and the Krebs cycle. Magnesium is also needed to stabilize ATP after it is produced, making it critical to any cellular function that relies on ATP. We produce our body weight in ATP molecules every day, but without magnesium, these ATP molecules are biologically useless. It also helps to relax muscles and regulate the nervous system, preventing over-stimulation of nerve cells.

Because it is so important to so many metabolic functions, the body raids its magnesium stores in response to stress. For example, stress hormones such as cortisol and adrenaline tend to mobilize magnesium to help produce extra ATP, contract muscles, and support the nervous system. Magnesium's involvement becomes even more critical during *oxidative* stress, especially when iron-catalyzed reactions are involved, as the heart and other metabolically active tissues use magnesium to repair oxidative damage.

As Robbins puts it, "all of the negative stressors we experience in our day to day lives become oxidative stress inside our cells, and

---

141 J.R. Conner and A.J. Ghio (As cited in Eugene D. Weinberg, "The Hazards of Iron Loading," *Metallomics* 2, no. 11 (2010): 732.)

142 Damiano Piovesan et al., "The Human 'Magnesome': Detecting Magnesium Binding Sites on Human Proteins," *BMC Bioinformatics* 13, no. S14 (September 2012).

oxidative stress eats magnesium for lunch."[143] This vivid analogy highlights the voracious consumption of magnesium during periods of stress, underscoring why magnesium deficiency is so widespread and its impact on energy production and antioxidant defenses so profound.

Finally, while iron overload drives oxidative stress and inflammation, and magnesium buffers against these processes by supporting energy production and cellular stability, copper emerges as the third key mineral in this trio, playing a vital yet often overlooked role in maintaining metabolic balance.

Copper is so vital that each mitochondrion contains a reservoir of about 50,000 copper atoms to support its functions. This mineral's unique ability to regulate both oxygen and iron—two highly reactive yet essential elements—makes it essential for controlling oxidative stress and enabling efficient aerobic energy production.

Copper's Ability to Regulate Oxygen. Copper plays a critical role in facilitating clean energy production within the mitochondria. Several complexes that make up the ETC depend on copper, with the final complex—where oxygen attracts electrons and pairs with hydrogen to form water—being particularly dependent on it. Breakdown of this complex allows electrons to leak from the chain, creating ROS in the mitochondria. Even when this happens, copper remains essential to help clean up the mess by supporting mitochondrial antioxidants (i.e., superoxide dismutase).

Copper's Ability to Regulate Iron. Copper is also critical for helping to regulate iron, preventing it from accumulating in tissues and engaging in harmful reactions with oxygen. This regulation is mediated by ceruloplasmin, a critical iron-transporting protein that absolutely requires copper to function properly. Copper enables ceruloplasmin to convert ferrous iron (Fe^{2+})—a more reactive and potentially harmful form—into ferric iron (Fe^{3+}), which is safer and can be incorporated into circulating proteins. This conversion is crucial for keeping iron in

---

143 Robbins, *Cu-RE Your Fatigue.*

circulation and minimizing oxidative stress-inducing reactions such as the Fenton reaction.

Maintaining the proper balance of these three key minerals—iron, magnesium, and copper—is essential to prevent widespread oxidation and inflammation. Iron, while necessary for oxygen transport, becomes dangerous when it accumulates and triggers oxidation. Magnesium, which is critical for combating stress and maintaining cellular stability, helps mitigate this oxidative stress. Copper, by regulating both oxygen and iron, limits the oxidative damage caused by excess iron and reduces the strain on magnesium stores.

In the next couple chapters, we'll discuss ways in which our diet participates in this balance.

One Root, Many Branches

Metabolic dysfunction is akin to the stem cell of disease. Just as a stem cell can differentiate into any of the body's more than 200 cell types, metabolic dysfunction—fundamentally a cellular issue—can manifest as a wide array of chronic diseases that plague humanity today. We've already touched on how various chronic conditions are deeply tied to metabolic health. To further explore and solidify this connection, let's examine two increasingly prevalent issues: mental disorders and infertility.

Mental Disorders and Metabolic Dysfunction

Mental clarity is foundational to a flourishing Christian life. Jesus emphasizes this in the first and greatest commandment: "Love the Lord your God with all your heart and with all your soul and with all your mind" (Matt. 22:37–38). Yet, as mental health issues have skyrocketed in recent decades, conventional treatments often fail to address the root causes, focusing instead on pharmaceutical interventions that, at best, reduce the severity of symptoms.

For example, depression was long attributed to a simple chemical imbalance, specifically a lack of serotonin, which could be treated by artificially boosting serotonin with selective serotonin reuptake inhibitors (SSRIs). These drugs became the cornerstone of clinical guidelines, with lifestyle interventions being considered "complementary alternative treatments." However, the decades-long reliance on SSRIs was challenged by a landmark study that debunked the "chemical imbalance" theory. The study found that SSRIs were no more effective than a placebo for about 85 percent of people, while often causing significant side effects.[144] A similar study found that exercise was about one and a half times as effective as a combination of psychotherapy and medication for depressed patients.[145]

Mental health disorders, while varied and complex, are often explicitly tied to metabolic dysfunction. Consider this: for every one-unit increase in the triglyceride-to-HDL ratio—a fundamental marker of metabolic health that should be kept as low as possible—people are 89 percent more likely to develop depression![146]

Dr. Chris Palmer, a faculty member at Harvard Medical School, formalized this connection in his "Brain Energy" theory, which links every symptom of every mental illness to cellular function.[147] According to his theory, impaired mitochondrial activity in brain cells leads to overactive, underactive, or absent brain functions. These disruptions are shaped by metabolic regulators such as epigenetics, hormones, neurotransmitters, and inflammation—once again underscoring

---

144 Joanna Moncrieff, Robert E. Cooper, Tom Stockmann, et al. "The Serotonin Theory of Depression: A Systematic Umbrella Review of the Evidence," *Molecular Psychiatry* 28 (2023): 3243–3256.

145 Bhupinder Singh, Timothy Olds, Rachel Curtis, et al. "Effectiveness of Physical Activity Interventions for Improving Depression, Anxiety, and Distress: An Overview of Systematic Reviews," *British Journal of Sports Medicine* 57, no. 9 (2023): 1203–1209.

146 Yvonne T. van der Feltz-Cornelis, et al., "Incident Major Depressive Disorder Predicted by Three Measures of Insulin Resistance: A Dutch Cohort Study," *American Journal of Psychiatry* 178, no. 10 (2021): 914–920, https://doi.org/10.1176/appi.ajp.2021.20101479.

147 For more on Dr. Palmer's work, see Christopher M. Palmer, *Brain Energy: A Revolutionary Breakthrough in Understanding Mental Health and Improving Treatment for Anxiety, Depression, OCD, PTSD, and More,* (New York: BenBella Books, 2022).

the interconnectedness of the body and the transformative potential of lifestyle interventions to improve metabolic health and mental well-being.

Infertility and Metabolic Dysfunction

In the same vein, infertility—now reaching epidemic proportions—presents a deeply personal challenge for many couples, including those in the Church. Scripture highlights several infertile women as testimonies to God's sovereignty and miraculous grace. Yet even though the Lord is said to open and close the womb,[148] the degree to which we participate by preparing our bodies is often downplayed in the modern health model, as is the strong influence of metabolic health.

In women, polycystic ovary syndrome (PCOS) is the leading cause of infertility.[149] This condition, marked by disruptions in sex hormones, interferes with ovulation and often results in irregular or absent menstrual cycles. Two key statistics underscore its metabolic roots: more than 50 percent of women with PCOS are also diagnosed with type 2 diabetes by age 40,[150] and PCOS can often be reversed through lifestyle interventions that restore metabolic health.[151] This means that metabolic dysfunction is often the root cause of infertility in women—a fact that conventional treatment approaches, focused on synthetic hormone therapy and invasive procedures, tend to overlook.

Although several hormones are involved in PCOS, insulin resistance and elevated insulin levels are common underlying disturbances. Testosterone is a natural precursor to estrogen, but chronically high insulin can prompt the ovaries to overproduce testosterone while

---

148 1 Samuel 1:5–6; Genesis 30:22.

149 Reproductive Health. "Infertility: Frequently Asked Questions," May 15, 2024. https://www.cdc.gov/reproductive-health/infertility-faq/index.html.

150 Diabetes, "Diabetes and Polycystic Ovary Syndrome (PCOS)," May 15, 2024. https://www.cdc.gov/diabetes/risk-factors/pcos-polycystic-ovary-syndrome.html.

151 Antonio Paoli, Luca Mancin, Maria C. Giacona, et al. "Effects of a Ketogenic Diet in Overweight Women with Polycystic Ovary Syndrome," *Journal of Translational Medicine* 18 (2020): 104.

simultaneously impairing its conversion to estrogen. This leaves the body flooded with testosterone and seriously inhibits natural female hormone cycles.

Hormone imbalance, however, is only one dimension of female infertility. A more foundational influence may be mitochondrial function and oxidative stress. A human egg cell contains hundreds of thousands of mitochondria—an order of magnitude more than any other cell type—because the earliest stages of embryonic development depend entirely on the mother's stored mitochondrial energy. These mitochondria must function flawlessly to support maturation, fertilization, and the first days of cell division. When oxidative stress overwhelms them, mitochondrial DNA is damaged, ATP production falters, and the probability of successful conception diminishes sharply.

While infertility is often perceived as a women's issue, male infertility is almost as common—and the statistics are alarming. One landmark study revealed that sperm counts in men dropped by more than 50 percent between 1973 and 2018, with the decline accelerating in recent years.[152] While female fertility has been described as a "complicated orchestra of hormones, with insulin as the conductor," male infertility is more straightforward, typically tied to low testosterone, mitochondrial dysfunction in sperm cells, and poor blood flow. Each of these factors is, of course, strongly influenced by general metabolic health.

Obesity, for example, significantly reduces testosterone levels in men because fat cells contain aromatase, the same enzyme that converts testosterone to estrogen in women's ovaries. Insulin resistance doesn't inhibit aromatase activity in fat cells nearly to the extent that it does in the ovaries, so excess body fat continues to convert testosterone to estrogen at high rates.[153] Ben Bikman, a prominent metabolic researcher,

---

152 Hagai Levine et al., "Temporal Trends in Sperm Count: A Systematic Review and Meta-Regression Analysis of Samples Collected Globally in the 20th and 21st Centuries," *Human Reproduction Update* 29, no. 2 (2023): 157–176.

153 The aromatization of testosterone in fat cells produces a less potent form of estrogen than that which is produced in a women's ovaries. This lesser form is still enough to significantly alter the hormonal balance of an obese man, but the same effect in obese women is not significant enough to compensate for the lack of estrogen production in the ovaries.

humorously compares excess body fat in men to a "giant ovary" because of this effect.[154]

Another crucial factor is blood flow. Proper circulation is essential for reproductive health, and one of the most significant metabolic disruptors of vascular function is chronically elevated insulin. Excess insulin promotes inflammation, stiffens and damages blood vessels, and interferes with the enzymes that produce nitric oxide—a molecule vital for vasodilation and healthy cardiovascular function. Insulin resistance also increases oxidative stress within the endothelium, further impairing vessel elasticity and reducing nutrient delivery to reproductive tissues. When blood flow is compromised in these ways, fertility in both sexes is adversely affected.

Therefore, while metabolic dysfunction is not always the sole cause of infertility, it is a significant and increasingly common contributor to the condition. Addressing its root causes offers a powerful opportunity to improve fertility outcomes and restore reproductive health.

Christ, Our Consolation

As we have seen, disease foreshadows and ushers in the realm of death. Despite our efforts to will and promote health—obediently respecting our lives as a loan held in trust—the realm of death still comes for everyone. But even in the face of this harsh reality, is not Christ, who conquered death, our ultimate consolation?

Some suggest that the next frontier of health and science is the complete abolition of death, as if death were merely a technical problem to be solved by scientific advancement. But Dr. John Lennox, a renowned mathematician and Christian apologist, offers a powerful reminder to those who anticipate this reality: "You're too late; the problem of physical death was solved 20 centuries ago."

What Lennox emphasizes is the hope of eternal life through the death and resurrection of Christ. Perhaps the physical decay we

---

154   Benjamin Bikman, *Why We Get Sick: The Hidden Epidemic at the Root of Most Chronic Disease—and How to Fight It* (BenBella Books, 2020), 43.

experience on earth serves as a teacher, helping us to appreciate this gift more fully.

Barth eloquently illustrates this perspective with a uniquely Christian approach to disease:

"But what if sickness as the concrete form of weakness, of destruction, of the impairing of his strength and powers, of growing old and declining, is the hard actuality which ushers in this genuinely liberating insight? What if it is not only the forerunner and messenger of death and judgment, but also, concealed under this form, the witness to God's creative goodness, the forerunner and messenger of the eternal life which God has allotted and promised to the man who is graciously preserved and guided by Him within the confines of his time?"[155]

Therefore, the Christian's attitude toward illness and death should be twofold: it can and should be actively resisted, but its ultimate inevitability reveals liberating truths that guide us toward a life well lived in anticipation of redeemed bodies in eternity.

In the chapters to come, we'll look at how our diets contribute to the onset of metabolic dysfunction. How do the foods we eat damage our mitochondria, disrupt the balance of our gut microbiome, and lead to critical mineral imbalances? Just as importantly, we'll examine how dietary choices can prevent or even reverse these harmful processes.

Ultimately, the degree to which our diets support health depends on how much they appeal to the logic of God's design. Food, by its very nature, is meant to nourish and heal the body. The more we distort its purpose—turning it into something artificial, over-processed, or made in our own image—the more we invite decay and dysfunction into ourselves.

---

155 Barth, *Church Dogmatics*, 373.

7

Discerning Dining (The Culprits of Metabolic Dysfunction)

> *"We all want progress. But progress means getting nearer to the place where you want to be. And if you have taken a wrong turning, then to go forward does not get you any nearer. If you are on the wrong road, progress means doing an about-turn and walking back to the right road...*
> *I think that if you look at the present state of the world, it is pretty plain that humanity has been making some big mistakes. We are on the wrong road. And if that is so, we must go back. Going back is the quickest way on."*
>
> – C.S. Lewis, Mere Christianity

C.S. Lewis brilliantly observed that movement is progress only if it brings us closer to God's design. However, it is plainly observable, as he would say, that we have taken some wrong turns, especially when it comes to nutrition. In an age in which our scientific and technological capabilities are exponentially more advanced than those of previous generations, and in which tens of thousands of peer-reviewed nutritional studies are published annually, Western society demonstrates that we are paradoxically more confused about how to feed ourselves than were our sheepherding ancestors.

Faced with this reality, the first step in the right direction is to simply stop and turn around. Eliminating or significantly reducing consumption of the "foods" most likely to make us sick, fat, and depressed is just as important, if not more so, than replacing them with those that promote our flourishing.

While this list could certainly be expanded, we'll highlight four of the most common, insidious, and perhaps controversial foods, chemicals, and supplements that harm our metabolic health. We'll explore how they contribute to disease and begin to develop strategies for avoiding or replacing them in our diets—a topic we'll continue to explore in the next chapter.

Refined Carbohydrates

It's easy to underappreciate the profound implications of the Creation account's description of the earth "bringing forth" plants.[156] The mechanism behind this process remained unknown for much of human history. It was once widely believed that plants were literally made of soil, but this idea was challenged in the 1600s when scientists observed trees growing in pots and noticed that while the trees grew larger, the soil level remained unchanged. We now know that while soil channels vitamins and minerals, the bulk of a plant's material comes from water in the soil and carbon dioxide in the air, made possible by the process of photosynthesis.

Carbohydrates, the primary product of photosynthesis, are essentially carbon atoms (carbo-) attached to water molecules (-hydrate). Glucose, a simple sugar, is the basic carbohydrate that plants produce as an immediate source of energy.

But forward-thinking plants also consider the need to store energy for lean times, so they link thousands of glucose molecules hand-in-hand

---

156 Genesis 1: 11–13.

to form long strands of starch, a more efficient storage form of glucose.[157] Plants—and humans, for that matter—can't use starch directly, but both rely on the enzyme alpha-amylase to break it down into individual glucose molecules. This process begins rapidly—so quickly, in fact, that starchy foods like white bread begin to dissolve into glucose even before swallowing, leaving a sweet aftertaste.

While glucose is sweet, fructose, another simple sugar, is even sweeter. Many plants produce fructose and store it in their fruit to entice animals to eat it and disperse their seeds. For even greater efficiency, plants condense glucose and fructose into sucrose, a compound that takes up less storage space than the two sugars separately.

All plants and plant-based foods contain a mix of these carbohydrates. Potatoes and pasta, for example, are almost entirely starch, while fruits are lower in starch and higher in simple sugars like fructose, glucose, and sucrose. The most important thing to understand about carbohydrates, though, is that all non-fibrous carbs—whether from a sweet treat like chocolate cake or a savory baked potato—are ultimately broken down into simple sugars in the bloodstream.[158]

In Scripture, sweetness is often used as a metaphor for holiness. The Psalmist writes, "How sweet are your words to my taste, sweeter than honey to my mouth!" (Ps. 119:103). Just as we need God's Word for spiritual nourishment, we need some sugar in our blood—described earlier as one form of "metabolic cash"—to feed our mitochondria.[159]

However, too much of a good thing can be a bad thing, especially when it comes to sugar. Glucose, a very sticky molecule, globs on to other molecules in the bloodstream through a process called glycation. This reaction produces advanced glycation end products (AGEs), aptly named for their key role in the aging process. Similar to the Maillard

---

157   Starch is essentially the same as glycogen, the body's short-term storage form of glucose.

158   For this reason, the effective "sugar" content of a food is often more than what is listed as sugar on the nutrition label. The real value can be calculated by subtracting the fiber content from the total carbohydrate content.

159   While fat can supply much of the body's energy demands (especially during fasting), glucose is still a preferred source of energy for many bodily functions.

reaction that browns toast, glycation "browns" proteins in the body, damaging collagen, elastin, and other essential structures over time. But AGEs do more than contribute to aging; they also drive chronic oxidative stress and inflammation—two key factors, as we've extensively discussed, that fuel metabolic dysfunction.[160]

No biological molecule is safe from glycation. Proteins, lipids, and even blood cells can be damaged, rendered dysfunctional, or prevented from reaching their destinations.

Collagen, the protein responsible for the structure and flexibility of blood vessels, is particularly vulnerable. Unlike lipids and blood cells, which are regularly renewed, collagen is more permanently affected. Glycated collagen stiffens over time, leading to hardened blood vessels—a major contributor to cardiovascular disease.[161]

More alarmingly, these cardiovascular effects, while significant, may pale in comparison to the impact of excess sugar on the brain, where it contributes to cognitive decline, neurodegenerative diseases, and mental health challenges.[162]

Earlier, we examined how our metabolic energy management system regulates blood glucose, maintaining just enough for immediate energy needs while avoiding excess. The damaging effects of glycation underscore why this regulation is so critical.

Although our metabolic energy management system is robust and capable of handling large carbohydrate loads, it is wise to eat in a way that minimizes the strain on it—particularly through carbohydrate management. Ideally, blood glucose levels should remain relatively stable, with gentle rises around meals rather than dramatic spikes and crashes—going wildly above baseline and then crashing below it. It's

---

160 J. Liu, S. Pan, X. Wang, et al., "Role of Advanced Glycation End Products in Diabetic Vascular Injury: Molecular Mechanisms and Therapeutic Perspectives," *European Journal of Medical Research* 28 (2023): 553.

161 Ibid.

162 A. Jacques, N. Chaaya, K. Beecher, S. A. Ali, A. Belmer, S. Bartlett, *The Impact of Sugar Consumption on Stress-Driven, Emotional and Addictive Behaviors,* Neurosci Biobehav Rev. 2019; 103: 178–199.

these frequent or extreme blood sugar swings that wreak havoc in the bloodstream and should be avoided through thoughtful dietary choices.

Tracking Glycation

Understanding glycation begins with monitoring blood glucose levels. A simple fasting blood glucose test is a rudimentary yet helpful gauge for understanding the body's glucose setpoint. While it shows up on a standard blood panel, a more frequent finger prick can help assess average levels over time. Anywhere between 70 and 85 mg/dL is considered optimal,[163] and consistent readings above this should be paired with an insulin test to determine the extent of insulin resistance in the body.

For a more detailed picture, a continuous glucose monitor (CGM) offers real-time insights into the body's blood sugar regulation throughout the day. By tracking fluctuations, a CGM not only highlights baseline fasting levels, but also visualizes spikes after meals, revealing how effectively the body is using insulin to manage glucose.

Finally, because the long-term effects of glycation are what matter most, the Hemoglobin A1c (HbA1c) test is an invaluable tool. HbA1c measures the percentage of glycated red blood cells and provides an average of glucose levels over the past 120 days. Lower results are better, as they indicate reduced glycation. While an HbA1c below 5.7 percent is considered normal, optimal levels are below 5.4 percent.

Fortunately, we can manage our blood sugar more easily by consuming carbohydrates according to nature's patterns.

Among the most notable of these patterns is that sweet foods are generally packaged with fiber, a complex carbohydrate that, although

---

163 The normal fasting blood glucose level is typically defined as up to 99 mg/dL, but it's important to approach "normal" values with caution and not confuse them with optimal levels for health. Metabolic dysfunction is the norm in modern society, so values that don't necessarily trigger an abnormal reading may still indicate an underlying issue.

made of glucose, isn't absorbed by the body as sugar. This simple fact is a part of God's divine logic. This fiber slows digestion, dampens blood sugar spikes, and helps insulin manage the influx of glucose. It also promotes satiety and aids digestion, topics we'll explore further in the next chapter.

But mankind, in its fallen ingenuity, has found ways to strip away the fiber, concentrating the sugar and distorting God's intended design. Highly refined sugars and grains—such as table sugar, fruit juices, syrups, white flour, and instant oats—dominate the Western diet, their harmful effects obscured by clever tactics and misconceptions propagated by the food industry and its allies.

Sugar's Disguises and Misconceptions

Hidden Sugars. One common tactic is to smuggle sugar into unexpected foods under one of more than 60 aliases, such as dextrose, maltose, evaporated cane juice, rice syrup, or barley malt. But no matter what seemingly wholesome term is used to disguise a carbohydrate's identity, the body processes these sugars in much the same way.

"Added" Sugars. Another widespread myth is the distinction between "added" and "naturally occurring" sugars—such as the sugars in an apple versus those in a jar of applesauce. Our bodies aren't fooled by this arbitrary distinction. Whether the sugar is added during processing or occurs naturally, it's the total sugar content—and what's been removed from the original food—that matters most. While added sugars are rightly scrutinized, even the original sugars can be problematic when separated from the fiber, water, and nutrients that normally accompany them.

For instance, dark chocolate, sweetened with a small amount of added sugar, offers health benefits due to its antioxidants and fats that slow sugar absorption. In contrast, apple juice, often marketed as free of added sugar, is essentially type 2 diabetes in a glass, offering virtually no benefits that would distinguish it from a can of soda. Even without *added* sugar, the *removal* of fiber concentrates the sugar and speeds its absorption in the body. While few people would consider eating more than one apple at a time, it's quite easy to guzzle a couple apples' worth of sugar in a glass of juice, which acts as a blunt and immediate infusion into the bloodstream.[164]

"Natural" Sugars. Similarly, the idea that "natural" sugars like honey, molasses, or maple syrup are inherently healthier than table sugar is misleading. But, again, this distinction is largely arbitrary; even table sugar comes from a plant and is therefore "natural" in some sense. While unrefined honey may have some beneficial compounds (depending on the source), we shouldn't assume that we can load up on "natural" sweeteners any more than the alternative; they all have a similar effect on the body's blood sugar levels, which is what *really* matters.

The "Low Glycemic" Fallacy. The final carbohydrate myth that leads us down the path to metabolic dysfunction is the notion that low-glycemic sweeteners—those with less impact on blood glucose levels—are inherently healthy. With our appreciation for blood sugar management, it would seem that sweeteners like agave nectar—extremely sweet and with a low glycemic index—would live up to the hype. Despite the allure, however, agave and similar plants are only low in glucose because they are extremely high in fructose! In other words, while they might not raise blood *glucose* levels very much, they still deliver a massive *fructose* load, which is far worse.

The Hidden Dangers of Fructose

While we typically think of blood sugar in terms of glucose (the sugar that insulin regulates), fructose behaves very differently in the body. The sweetest simple sugar, found naturally in fruits and added in concentrated form to many processed foods, fructose is even stickier

---

164 This is the fatal flaw of the juicing trend, which does nothing but remove the fiber and concentrate the sugar. For this reason, a counterintuitive trend known as "reverse juicing" has gained some traction. As the name implies, reverse juicing involves extracting the juice from fruits and vegetables, but instead of drinking the juice and tossing the fibrous pulp, people consume the pulp and toss the juice.

than glucose, making it 10 times more likely to cause glycation (and thus AGE-ing)!

Because it comes primarily from fruit, fructose is naturally most abundant in the fall and signals the body to fatten up for winter by turning off its satiety signals. What's more, while glucose can be used for energy by almost every cell in the body, fructose is processed almost exclusively by the liver, where it is either used for energy or turned into fat.

For this reason, fructose has been known to cause non-alcoholic fatty liver disease since ancient times.[165] In fact, the first-century Roman chef Marcus Apicius used this knowledge to perfect his recipe for foie gras, or goose liver. His ingenious technique for fattening the livers of his geese involved feeding them large quantities of dates (high in fructose).

According to the ancient historian Pliny the Elder,

"Apicius made the discovery, that we may employ the same artificial method of increasing the size of the liver of the sow, as of that of the goose; it consists in cramming them with dried figs, and when they are fat enough, they are drenched with wine mixed with honey, and immediately killed."[166]

So while it's important, especially for diabetics, to monitor blood glucose levels and avoid glucose spikes, we shouldn't overlook fructose, which is invisible to these metrics, but quite harmful when concentrated and consumed in large quantities.[167]

This revelation about fructose adds a wrinkle to our understanding of carbohydrates. Although all non-fibrous carbohydrates ultimately enter the bloodstream as simple sugars, the type of simple sugar makes a difference. For example, 50 grams of carbohydrate from chocolate

---

165 Thomas Jensen et al., "Fructose and Sugar: A Major Mediator of Non-Alcoholic Fatty Liver Disease," *Journal of Hepatology* 68, no. 5 (2018): 1063–1075.

166 Pliny the Elder (as cited in Jensen et al., "Fructose and Sugar: A Major Mediator of Non-Alcoholic Fatty Liver Disease").

167 This is another reason why it's important to measure HbA1c periodically, as it measures total glycation (from fructose and glucose), as opposed to other glucose-centric measures, like blood sugar.

cake—mostly sucrose (equal parts glucose and fructose)—is more taxing than 50 grams of starch from French fries—all of which is broken down into glucose.

Restoring a Healthy Relationship with Carbs

Carbohydrates aren't the devil incarnate, but they are certainly among his favorite tools for making us fat, sick, and depressed. In C.S. Lewis's *The Screwtape Letters*, the senior demon Screwtape instructs his nephew, Wormwood, on the subtle ways to corrupt the human soul, alluding to humanity's affinity for sweets as a potential weakness to be exploited. We now know that this propensity doesn't just affect our souls; it degrades our hearts, brains, and overall metabolic health.

Lewis's insight reveals how our misuse of sugar reflects a deeper aspect of our fallen nature. We often misappropriate God's gifts—meant for nourishment and joy—in ways that harm us and distort their intended purpose. Instead of receiving them with gratitude and restraint, we consume them compulsively, severed from the logic of God's design. Nevertheless, it's possible—and practical—to restore a healthy relationship with carbohydrates. That begins by understanding how our bodies process them: the damaging effects of glycation, the different metabolic paths of glucose and fructose, and the role of insulin in managing both. When we grasp these mechanisms, we can more clearly identify misleading labels, resist fads that demonize or glorify the wrong things, and avoid sugar in its most stripped, concentrated forms.

Is Bread Off-Limits?

We explored the anthropological significance of bread back in Chapter Two, finding it to be the preeminent symbol of human nourishment (at least for fallen humanity) and, most importantly, the food Christ would eventually choose to represent His own body. But what about all those carbs?

Bread has earned a bad reputation in modern nutritional advice—and not without reason. Most commercial bread is made from highly refined wheat, where the nutrient-rich bran and germ are stripped away, leaving only the starchy endosperm. This process extends shelf life but removes much of the fiber, vitamins, minerals, and healthy fats that make whole grains nourishing. Even so-called "whole wheat" bread is often highly processed, with the parts separated, ground finely, and reconstituted—giving the appearance of wholesomeness while offering little of its original integrity.

But this kind of bread is essentially a modern invention (some might even say an abomination). Traditionally, flour was freshly milled, preserving the full nutritional glory of the wheat berry and yielding a more complex, slowly digesting carbohydrate along with essential nutrients like vitamin E, B vitamins, magnesium, and healthy fats. Sue Becker, a Christian food scientist, baker, and passionate advocate for real bread, argues that if we simply returned to this time-honored practice—perhaps with the help of a modern electric grain mill—we could recover a wheat bread that not only tastes better but is genuinely good for us. Indeed, even many people with autoimmune conditions or gluten sensitivities report that this kind of bread isn't just tolerable, but often healing.

So, is bread off-limits? Certainly not! But it's wise to avoid store-bought varieties and consider returning to a time more like that described in Deuteronomy 24:6, when the family mill was central to daily life.

A healthy relationship with carbs, however, doesn't necessarily mean avoiding even refined carbohydrates entirely. For most of us, there will be times when we want to indulge in a bowl of refined pasta or a slice (or two) of sugary apple pie. And while these aren't the kinds of foods to build a diet on, there are practical ways to temper such occasional indulgences. Consider the tradition of starting a meal with a salad. This may be more than just cultural habit; eating fiber-rich foods first helps trap sugars during digestion, reducing the spike in blood glucose and insulin. The same carbohydrate load causes less damage when its release is slowed. A vinegar-based dressing can enhance this effect, as vinegar slows gastric emptying and improves insulin sensitivity, promoting a more stable metabolic response.[168]

It's also wise to avoid eating "naked carbs"—carbohydrates consumed without accompanying fat, fiber, or protein. These bare sugars digest rapidly and flood the bloodstream, spiking insulin and increasing the risk of fat storage and energy crashes. Adding healthy fats, protein, or fibrous vegetables to a carbohydrate-rich food can significantly blunt this effect and better align with the body's natural regulatory systems.

Moderate physical activity immediately before or after a meal can further improve the body's ability to dispose of glucose. A short walk, fifteen push-ups, or ten air squats can dramatically reduce post-meal blood sugar spikes for many people. The growing use of continuous glucose monitors has validated these strategies, empowering individuals to experiment and discover what helps them enjoy sweetness without sacrificing metabolic health in a broken food culture.[169]

To conclude this section, it's worth pointing out that carbohydrates are the only non-essential macronutrient: our bodies can manufacture all the glucose they need from protein or fat, so we don't have to eat carbs to stay alive. Still, let's be honest—life is richer, meals are more satisfying, and physical performance often improves when wholesome carbohydrates are on the table. The key is discernment. Carbohydrates—especially those from fruit, vegetables, "real" bread, and raw honey—should be enjoyed with a clear grasp of how they work in the body, how much is appropriate for a given activity level, and how highly refined alternatives can become a snare that distorts our relationship with them.

---

168 C. S. Johnston, et al., "Vinegar Improves Insulin Sensitivity to a High-Carbohydrate Meal in Subjects with Insulin Resistance or Type 2 Diabetes," *Diabetes Care* 27, no. 1 (2004): 281–82.

169 For more information on some of the most effective strategies for managing blood sugar levels, refer to *The Glucose Revolution* by Jessie Inchauspé.

Ultra-Processed Oils

Most people are aware that there are "good" fats and "bad" fats, but while this distinction is real, it may be along a different line than the mainstream consensus suggests. Proverbs 14:12 warns, "There is a way that seems right to a man, but its end is the way to death." This verse underscores the contrast between God's perfect wisdom and our flawed human judgment—a theme echoed in our treatment of dietary fats. Nature, embedded with the divine Logos, does not produce inherently "bad" fats, as we'll continue to explore in the next chapter. The focus of this section, however, is how human intervention has altered certain fats in ways that contribute to disease and even death, reflecting the proverb's caution.

These harmful fats come primarily in the form of cheap, ultra-processed oils. A cornerstone of the ultra-processed food industry, they appear in almost every pantry staple, baked good, and fried food. Some of the most common offenders are mayonnaise, salad dressing, peanut butter, margarine, non-dairy creamers, cookies, French fries, pizza, chips, and the list goes on and on. Even many so-called "health foods," such as hummus and pesto, feature these oils toward the top of their ingredients list. Ironically, even the "organic" label—intended to signal natural, minimally-processed origins—doesn't exclude ultra-processed oils.

Yet, despite their ubiquity and general acceptance, these oils tend to be masked by misleading labels. For example, they're often called "vegetable oils," suggesting a wholesome origin like broccoli or carrots. They're also called "seed oils," but not all problematic oils come from seeds, nor are all seed-derived oils unhealthy. For example, sesame oil—a traditional staple in Eastern cuisine—is relatively harmless, while soybean oil is far from benign.

Dr. Cate Shanahan, a leading expert on the dangers of these ultra-processed oils, identifies eight that should be avoided like the plague, dubbing them the "Hateful Eight": canola, corn, and cottonseed oils (the "Three Cs"); sunflower, safflower, and soybean oils (the "Three Ss"); grapeseed; and rice bran.

The rise of these oils to dietary prominence reflects an unfortunate convergence of industrialization, economic policy, and misguided medical advice.

The Rise of Ultra-Processed Oils

Historically, culinary traditions relied on animal fats such as lard, tallow, and butter. But while flavorful and effective, their perishable nature and higher cost led to a decline in popularity during the early twentieth century. As the Industrial Revolution progressed, chemists found ways to extract oils from seeds and other abundant plant materials, often repurposing waste byproducts such as cottonseed from the cotton industry. These oils were cheap and shelf stable, but initially failed to gain traction as food products, in large part because they didn't taste very good.

The World Wars played a key role in their adoption, as animal fats were rationed, making these oils a practical, even patriotic, alternative. But they weren't all used for food. In fact, soybean and cottonseed oils became commodities because of their effective use as machine lubricants, soaps, and paints. After World War II, massive government subsidies and agricultural advancements created surpluses of soybeans, corn, and similar crops, leading to an abundant supply of oils derived from them.

However, despite advances in processing technology and an abundance of source crops, these oils didn't become dietary staples until saturated fats were controversially linked to cholesterol and heart disease—a connection we'll examine in the next chapter. Once it was established that they could lower cholesterol, all commercial manufacturers had to do was reduce their stench, make them bland in flavor, and secure the American Heart Association's stamp of approval, turning them into ubiquitous pantry essentials and a cornerstone of the processed food industry.

But unlike their natural predecessors, consuming these oils is like drinking a bottle of oxidation and inflammation soup. This stark difference lies in their chemical composition, which plays a key role in how they interact with our bodies.

The Chemistry (and Consequences) of Fats

Fats are long chains of fatty acids held together by carbon bonds. Each carbon bond in these fatty acid chains is "saturated" when it is completely filled with hydrogen atoms. Therefore, if a carbon bond is missing a pair of hydrogens, the bond is said to be unsaturated, resembling a flexible "kink" in the fatty acid chain.

Saturated Fats. Saturated fats have no double carbon bonds, which makes their chains rigid and straight (without any "kinks"). For this reason, they are typically solid at room temperature, as seen in butter.

Monounsaturated Fats. These fatty acids have a single double carbon bond, giving them a "kink" that keeps them liquid at room temperature but solid when refrigerated, like olive oil.

Polyunsaturated Fats (PUFAs). PUFAs have more than one unsaturated bond, with the added flexibility evident in their low melting point, which keeps them liquid even in the refrigerator (think commercial salad dressings). PUFAs are especially abundant in plants from colder climates, where lower melting points help their seeds germinate in cool spring soils.

The most important thing to understand about the Hateful Eight ultra-processed oils is that they are derived from predominantly cold weather plants and are thus largely made of PUFAs. The problem, however, is that the highly flexible and unsaturated structures of these fatty acids leave many openings for oxygen molecules to squeeze in, making them uniquely prone to damage via oxidation.

Despite their instability, PUFAs aren't inherently harmful. In fact, they are critical to our survival—at least in small amounts. Both omega-3 and omega-6 fatty acids, the two major categories of PUFAs, play crucial roles in the body and are considered essential fatty acids, meaning they cannot be synthesized by the body and must be obtained through diet. When left in their natural state, such as in seeds or nuts, their inherent instability is offset by protective antioxidants and other beneficial compounds, which is why whole sunflower seeds, for instance, are quite nutritious.

The problem arises when the oil is extracted, stripping away these protective compounds and exposing the PUFAs to oxidation. Traditional oils like olive, avocado, or macadamia nut oil come from plants that naturally produce oil-rich fruits or nuts, which can be cold-pressed to preserve their flavors and protective elements. Good luck attempting to extract cottonseed oil or soybean oil in this wholesome manner. These oils are ultra-processed for a reason: there's no other way to get them out.

Omega-3 and-6 PUFAs

The "omega" number in a PUFA refers to the position of the first double bond, or "kink," in the carbon chain, counted from the methyl (omega) end. In omega-3 fatty acids this first double bond is located at the third carbon from the end, and likewise for omega-6 fatty acids. This structural variation greatly influences the unique properties and functions of each type of fatty acid.

Omega-3 fatty acids are celebrated for their anti-inflammatory properties and are essential for brain health, cellular stability, and cardiovascular health. Common sources include fatty fish, flaxseed, and walnuts. Omega-6 fatty acids, on the other hand, are essential for skin health and cell membrane flexibility. While they are inherently pro-inflammatory, this property is critical for supporting the immune response to injury and infection. Omega-6 is abundant in most nuts, seeds, and ultra-processed oils.

Because omega-3 and omega-6 fatty acids have opposing roles in inflammation, maintaining a balanced ratio is essential for optimal health. Historically, this ratio was roughly 1:1. However, the modern diet—where ultra-processed oils make up about 10 percent of daily caloric intake[170]—has skewed this ratio closer to 15:1.[171] This imbalance is thought to independently contribute to widespread chronic inflammation and exacerbate the negative health effects of ultra-processed oils.[172]

The extraction process for these oils begins by subjecting the seeds or plant material to high heat and intense mechanical pressing to release some of the oil. The remaining "oil cake" is then treated with chemical solvents, such as hexane, to dissolve any remaining oil. At this stage, the crude oil has a repulsive flavor and odor, so no one would mistake it for a food product. It must still undergo extensive refining to make it remotely palatable. This refining process includes degumming, neutralizing, washing, drying, bleaching (to remove color), dewaxing, and finally deodorizing at high temperatures to eliminate any remaining flavors.[173] By the end of this process, the oil has been stripped of its original protective plant compounds and pulverized with oxygen, creating a highly unstable cocktail of free radicals.

Because they are affectionately known as "cooking oils," the damage continues when they are used in a frying pan or—God forbid—in a McDonald's deep fryer, sometimes for several days. Heating, especially repeated heating, further amplifies the formation of inflammatory compounds. For example, just one gram of oxidized frying oil can deliver five times the WHO's estimated upper daily limit for toxic aldehydes—meaning that a single basket of French fries, which can

170 James J. DiNicolantonio and James H. O'Keefe. "Omega-6 Vegetable Oils as a Driver of Coronary Heart Disease: The Oxidized Linoleic Acid Hypothesis." *Open Heart* 5 (2018): e000898.

171 Artemis P. Simopoulos, "Evolutionary Aspects of Diet, the Omega-6/Omega-3 Ratio and Genetic Variation: Nutritional Implications for Chronic Diseases," *Biomedicine & Pharmacotherapy* 60, no. 9 (2006): 502–507.

172 James J. DiNicolantonio and James H. O'Keefe, "Importance of Maintaining a Low Omega–6/Omega–3 Ratio for Reducing Inflammation," *Open Heart* 5 (2018): e000946.

173 Said Gharby, "Refining Vegetable Oils: Chemical and Physical Refining," *The Scientific World Journal* 2022 (January 11, 2022): 6627013.

absorb 10 to 20 grams of oil, may deliver more than fifty times that threshold in one meal.[174]

But even when they aren't used for cooking, being used in salad dressings, mayonnaise, or other processed foods, these oils are poison for our mitochondria. Remember, oxygen is critical for energy production in our mitochondria, but PUFAs are volatile in the presence of oxygen. Unlike stable saturated fats, which act like high-octane, clean-burning fuel for our cells, injecting high concentrations of PUFAs into our mitochondria is like pumping low-grade gasoline into a sports car, causing knocking, incomplete combustion, and harmful residue buildup. In cellular terms, the result is reduced energy production, more oxidative stress, and impaired insulin signaling.

Recognizing the harm these oils cause *within* the body—promoting inflammation and destabilizing energy production—is alarming enough. But even more disturbing is the extent to which these fats have become *part of* the body. Research shows that omega-6 PUFAs from ultra-processed oils have significantly accumulated in our adipose tissue, effectively changing the stuff we're made of. A 2015 review highlighted that PUFA levels in body fat have increased by about 2.5-fold over the past half century, a tangible reflection of our increased consumption of ultra-processed oils during this time.[175]

When these highly volatile compounds saturate our fat stores, they transform adipose tissue into what Dr. Cate Shanahan calls "sick fat," which behaves very differently from healthy fat and is a major contributor to insulin resistance. Specifically, fat cells with high concentrations of omega-6 linoleic acid tend to stop multiplying and instead grow larger. As they expand, they become stressed and begin to spill free fatty acids— an environment that invites pro-inflammatory macrophages. These

---

174 M. Grootveld, "Evidence-Based Challenges to the Continued Recommendation and Use of Peroxidatively-Susceptible Polyunsaturated Fatty Acid-Rich Culinary Oils for High-Temperature Frying Practises: Experimental Revelations Focused on Toxic Aldehydic Lipid Oxidation Products," Frontiers in Nutrition 8 (2022): 711640, https://doi.org/10.3389/fnut.2021.711640

175 Stephan J. Guyenet and Susan E. Carlson, "Increase in Adipose Tissue Linoleic Acid of US Adults in the Last Half Century," *Advances in Nutrition* 6, no. 6 (November 13, 2015): 660–664.

immune cells release cytokines that directly inhibit insulin signaling pathways, sowing the seeds of systemic insulin resistance. In short, sick fat behaves as though it were infected, belching inflammatory distress signals that promote widespread inflammation. When we build our bodies from volatile fats, we should not be surprised when metabolic dysfunction follows.

Ultra-processed oils are a modern "franken-food," unknown to the human diet until the twentieth century—and they have no rightful place in it now. Understandably, one might ask, "What should I do if my pantry is full of these cheap, ultra-processed oils?" The best—though perhaps most difficult—solution is to discard anything that contains canola, corn, cottonseed, sunflower, safflower, soybean, grapeseed, or rice bran oil. Do so with confidence and a clear conscience, knowing that these oils ceased to be a part of God's design for human flourishing when they were extracted in the first place. Ultimately, the temporary financial pinch of shifting away from ultra-processed foods pays a large and compounding dividend in the health bank account that promotes true, eternal wealth.

Herbicides and Pesticides

To understand why herbicides and pesticides pose such a pervasive threat, we must first take a high-level view of life on Earth. Chloroplasts—the microbial cousins of our mitochondria—are the organelles responsible for photosynthesis in plants, capturing sunlight and using its energy to convert CO_2 into sugars and fatty acids. This process effectively stores solar energy in the double carbon bonds of these molecules, which can later be released to fuel the activities of life. As discussed, our mitochondria do the hard work of breaking down these carbon bonds and releasing the sun's energy in the form of high-energy electrons, which are used in the ETC to produce ATP. God's wonderful design for life on earth is based on the ability of plants to capture sunlight and our cells (or the cells of the animals we consume) to convert it into usable energy.

The Ubiquity of Glyphosate in Modern Agriculture

However, this balance began to shift dramatically in the mid–twentieth century with the widespread adoption of synthetic chemical herbicides. Glyphosate, the active ingredient in Monsanto's Roundup herbicide, exemplifies this shift. Introduced in 1974, glyphosate targets the shikimate pathway—a critical system plants use to produce essential aromatic amino acids such as tryptophan, phenylalanine, and tyrosine. By inhibiting this pathway, glyphosate prevents plants from synthesizing key proteins, ultimately killing them.

Over the decades, Roundup became one of the most widely used herbicides in the world, particularly after the introduction in the 1990s of "Roundup Ready" genetically engineered crops such as corn, soybeans, cotton, and canola—engineered to resist glyphosate. Its use expanded not only for in-season weed control but also for pre-plant "burndown" applications and, in some regions and crops, limited pre-harvest desiccation to promote uniform drying. In sugarcane production, glyphosate has also been used as a chemical ripener to enhance sucrose accumulation under certain conditions.[176] Because of its broad-spectrum effectiveness, relatively low cost, and compatibility with large-scale mechanized farming, glyphosate use increased substantially over the past several decades. Today it is applied on hundreds of millions of acres globally each year. It is especially prevelant in conventional wheat-based products, oat-based foods, grain products, and legumes, and one nationally-representative study detected glyphosate in urine samples of 81% of Americans, with the highest levels in children.[177]

---

176 Anthony Samsel and Stephanie Seneff, "Glyphosate's Suppression of Cytochrome P450 Enzymes and Amino Acid Biosynthesis by the Gut Microbiome: Pathways to Modern Diseases," *Entropy* 15, no. 4 (2013): 1416–63.

177 Maria Ospina et al., "Exposure to Glyphosate in the United States: Data from the 2013–2014 National Health and Nutrition Examination Survey," *Environment International* 170 (2022)

Initially, concerns about glyphosate's impact on human health were minimal because plants, not animals, use the shikimate pathway that it targets. However, this assumption overlooked a crucial fact: bacteria and fungi also rely on the shikimate pathway! Glyphosate was originally patented as an antibiotic, underscoring its potency against these organisms. What Monsanto's engineers and federal regulators failed to consider is that the human body is host to a vast, intricate "organic garden" of bacteria and other microorganisms essential for health—making glyphosate's impact far more problematic than originally believed.

Health Impacts of Glyphosate

Stephanie Seneff, a leading expert on the health effects of glyphosate, has linked its rise in the food supply to a corresponding rise in conditions such as autism, obesity, kidney disease, celiac disease, cancer, neurological disorders, and a host of other ailments.[178] Several mechanisms are likely behind this toxic effect:

Glyphosate Chelates Minerals. By binding to trace elements like sulfur, selenium, and copper, glyphosate reduces the nutrient density of foods and deprives the human body of critical minerals. Roundup-treated crops are notably deficient in several key minerals, including sodium, sulfur, potassium, magnesium, and a variety of microminerals such as copper and boron. When consumed, glyphosate residues in food continue to chelate minerals in the human body, exacerbating deficiencies in copper and magnesium, both of which (as we explored) are critical for metabolic health.[179]

Glyphosate's Effect on Mitochondrial Function. Glyphosate's ability to disrupt mitochondrial function is also of concern. Roundup is known to disrupt mitochondrial ATP production, primarily by interfering with the electron transport chain. This disruption not only

---

178 Anthony Samsel and Stephanie Seneff, "Pathways to Modern Diseases" series, 2013, 2015, 2016, 2017.

179 Samsel and Seneff, "Glyphosate's Suppression of Cytochrome P450 Enzymes."

reduces the efficiency of energy production but also leads to electron leakage and the excessive production of ROS, resulting in oxidative stress.[180] As previously discussed, sluggish and damaged mitochondria are a major contributor to metabolic dysfunction.

Glyphosate's Impact on the Gut Microbiome. The other critical bugs in our bodies, those that inhabit our gut, are also profoundly affected by glyphosate. As a patented antibiotic, glyphosate significantly alters the composition of the gut microbiome. It selectively kills beneficial bacteria while allowing glyphosate-resistant pathogens to flourish. Widespread use of glyphosate selectively shifts the balance of the gut microbiome in favor of these pathogenic bacteria, many of which are known to produce pro-inflammatory cytokines and ROS. Some of these pathogens activate a signaling molecule called zonulin, which disrupts the tight junctions in the intestinal lining, leading to leaky gut.[181]

Moreover, glyphosate-sensitive bacteria are often those responsible for producing SCFAs and key amino acids like tryptophan and L-glutamate. These compounds are vital precursors to neurotransmitters that are critical for mental health and brain function.[182] To make matters worse, tryptophan is normally metabolized by these glyphosate-sensitive bugs, producing several additional compounds that protect against DNA damage and help prevent Alzheimer's disease.[183] For these reasons, glyphosate's impact on the composition of the gut microbiome certainly provides a link not only to leaky gut and inflammation, but also to

---

180 Olha M. Strilbytska et al., "The Effects of Low-Toxic Herbicide Roundup and Glyphosate on Mitochondria," *EXCLI Journal* 21 (January 2022): 183–96.

181 Alessio Fasano, "Zonulin and Its Regulation of Intestinal Barrier Function: The Biological Door to Inflammation, Autoimmunity, and Cancer," *Physiological Reviews* 91, no. 1 (2011): 151–75 (as cited in Samsel and Seneff, 2013).

182 Lauren Walsh et al., "Impact of Glyphosate (Roundup™) on the Composition and Functionality of the Gut Microbiome," *Gut Microbes* 15, no. 2 (2023): 2263935.

183 Linda S. Zhang and Sean S. Davies, "Microbial Metabolism of Dietary Components to Bioactive Metabolites: Opportunities for New Therapeutic Interventions," *Genome Medicine* 8, no. 1 (April 2016) (as cited in Gundry, *Gut Check*).

several neurological diseases often associated with altered gut flora, including Parkinson's,[184] schizophrenia,[185] and depression.[186]

Practical Steps to Minimize Exposure

With about one billion pounds of the stuff sprayed worldwide each year, avoiding exposure to pesticides and herbicides (especially glyphosate) altogether can be a challenge. However, there are simple guidelines for significantly reducing intake of these harmful chemicals.

One effective strategy is to choose organic foods. While this label has its flaws, organic produce is typically free of glyphosate and other synthetic chemicals common in conventional farming. While organic foods may be less accessible in some regions, occupy a smaller portion of the grocery store, and cost more than their non-organic counterparts, they are a safer choice for those seeking to reduce their glyphosate exposure.

But those unable or unwilling to go completely organic can at least make targeted choices by following the advice of the Environmental Working Group (EWG), which publishes an annual report that highlights pesticide contamination in produce. Their "Dirty Dozen" list identifies fruits and vegetables with the highest levels of pesticide residues, typically including strawberries, spinach, apples, and blueberries. These are the foods to either buy organic or not buy at all. On the other hand, EWG's "Clean 15" list features conventionally grown produce with the fewest pesticide residues, normally including

---

184 Erin M. Hill-Burns et al., "Parkinson's Disease and Parkinson's Disease Medications Have Distinct Signatures of the Gut Microbiome," *Movement Disorders* 32, no. 5 (February 2017): 739–49 (as cited in Gundry, *Gut Check*).

185 Tanya T. Nguyen et al., "Gut Microbiome in Serious Mental Illnesses: A Systematic Review and Critical Evaluation," *Schizophrenia Research* 234 (August 2021): 24–40 (as cited in Gundry, *Gut Check*).

186 Jian-jun Chen et al., "Sex Differences in Gut Microbiota in Patients With Major Depressive Disorder," *Neuropsychiatric Disease and Treatment* 14 (February 2018): 647–55 (as cited in Gundry, *Gut Check*).

avocados, onions, sweet potatoes, and carrots, giving a license to go cheap on these staples when necessary.

Misguided Micronutrients

Finally, the last major source of nutritional chaos may be a surprising one. Many people take nutritional supplements, especially multivitamins, out of concern that they aren't getting enough key micronutrients in their diets. This is a legitimate concern for most people, since our food is much less nutrient-dense than it used to be. But while micronutrient-dense foods should be a dietary priority (as we'll see in the next chapter) many commonly recommended vitamin and mineral supplements are misguided, with unintended metabolic consequences. Often, people aren't aware of the effects of synthetic or unnatural forms of micronutrients on critical balances in the body, such as the trio of minerals—iron, magnesium, and copper—introduced in the last chapter.[187]

Supplemental Iron

As we've already explored, iron is one of the most pro-oxidant metals on earth, and when it detaches from functional proteins and deposits in body tissues, it drives oxidative stress. Experts in iron metabolism agree that we aren't meant to store large amounts of iron but instead should maintain just enough for the metal's vital metabolic purposes, with little left over.

Nevertheless, iron supplementation is widespread. Multivitamins, prenatal vitamins, and fortified foods are loaded with it. According to Greek mythology, an ancient Persian physician prescribed sweet wine laced with iron filings to Jason and his crew of Argonauts as a form of body armor. Today's approach is hardly different. Since 1941, the U.S.

---

187 The following five supplements are inspired by the research of Morley Robbins, documented in his comprehensive "Root Cause Protocol" and in his book *Cu-RE Your Fatigue*.

has added inorganic iron filings to flour and grains to prevent anemia, increasing the dose by 50 percent in 1969.[188]

The truth, however, is that 95 percent of our needs should be met by recycling cellular iron, meaning that we need to consume only a few milligrams of iron per day—an amount readily available from unenriched foods.

So why the "fortification" frenzy?

The answer lies in a common confusion between iron *deficiency* and iron *dysregulation*. As Morley Robbins points out, many doctors mistakenly attribute anemia to low iron levels, but the real problem is usually dysfunctional iron metabolism. Rather than lacking iron, many people—especially in well-fed Western societies—struggle to use it properly. Functional iron requires the presence of other key nutrients like bioavailable copper and magnesium. Without these, iron is stored in tissues like the liver and heart, where it becomes harmful.

For this reason, most people should avoid supplemental iron, whether from multivitamins, prenatal supplements, or fortified foods. The only time to consider iron supplementation is after a comprehensive iron panel confirms a true deficiency, as interpreted by an iron-literate health professional.

Synthetic Vitamin C

Vitamin C is one of the most popular supplements, known for its antioxidant and immune-boosting properties. However, most "vitamin C" on the market is not real vitamin C, but synthetic ascorbic acid—a highly processed, test-tube chemical derived almost entirely from genetically modified Chinese corn. Unlike God's design for vitamin C, this isolated compound is incomplete and potentially harmful.

---

188   The USDA sought to triple the amount of iron enrichment in 1969, but settled for only a 50 percent increase due to warnings from several scientists. It's easy to spot these filings in food, as there is a classic experiment in which people crush Corn Flakes and run a magnet over them, finding that bits of the added iron collect on the magnet. These inorganic iron filings are far less biologically useful than iron bound to organic molecules, tending to deposit into bodily tissues.

If real vitamin C were a car, ascorbic acid would be its body, but without the engine, transmission, or steering wheel. True vitamin C contains bioflavonoids, lipids, enzymes, and other essential cofactors that make it biologically functional. One key component, the enzyme tyrosinase, is the "engine" of vitamin C, critical for protecting against UV rays and supporting the production of melanin—a pigment vital for skin, hair, eyes, and metabolic health. Synthetic ascorbic acid lacks this enzyme.

At best, synthetic ascorbic acid is incomplete and unworthy of the name vitamin C. At worst, it is harmful. Isolated ascorbic acid is much more acidic than natural vitamin C, which can interfere with copper absorption and degrade ceruloplasmin—a copper-based protein essential for regulating iron.[189]

For these reasons, it's best to avoid synthetic ascorbic acid, which is often added to processed foods, beverages, and multivitamins. True vitamin C—found in whole foods such as fruits and vegetables—works as part of a complete system designed to nourish and protect the body. In the next chapter, we'll explore the importance of getting biologically complete vitamin C from whole food sources.

Supplemental Vitamin D

In the early twenty-first century, vitamin D_3 supplements surged in popularity after public health officials declared a global deficiency and linked low levels of vitamin D to inflammation and chronic disease.[190] This guidance intensified during the COVID-19 pandemic, with health officials urging people to pop vitamin D pills as if their lives depended on it. But unlike most nutrients, vitamin D is not primarily obtained from food, with fatty fish being one of the few natural sources. Instead, the human body is designed to synthesize vitamin D through sun

---

189   The Root Cause Protocol, "FAQ - Whole Food Vitamin C vs Ascorbic Acid - The Root Cause Protocol," April 2, 2024, https://therootcauseprotocol.com/faq-whole-food-vitamin-c/.

190   Meg Mangin et al., "Inflammation and Vitamin D: The Infection Connection," *Inflammation Research* 63, no. 10 (July 2014): 803–19.

exposure, which not only produces sufficient amounts, but also adjusts our metabolism to seasonal changes—a benefit that indiscriminate pill-popping cannot replicate.

There are several reasons why the standard advice to boost vitamin D levels through supplementation is not only misguided, but perhaps even harmful:

Supplemental D Depletes Magnesium. Supplemental vitamin D (calcidiol) differs from the active form (calcitriol) produced by sun exposure. Converting calcidiol to calcitriol is a taxing load that requires both energy and several magnesium-dependent enzymes. For this reason, supplemental vitamin D saps magnesium levels in the body.

Supplemental D Depletes Potassium. One of the primary functions of vitamin D is to facilitate the absorption of calcium. In excess, this calcium can calcify cardiovascular soft tissues, contributing to heart disease. It also exacerbates magnesium consumption, as magnesium is a key regulator of calcium. Most alarmingly, however, the kidneys must excrete potassium to balance this mineral load, a serious condition called "potassium wasting."[191] This loss of potassium impairs the body's ability to regulate blood pressure and stress, leading to a cascade of metabolic consequences.

Supplemental D Disrupts Vitamin A Balance. Vitamins D and A work together in nature, balancing each other in animal-based foods like liver, egg yolks, and cod liver oil. For example, while vitamin D enhances calcium absorption, vitamin A ensures that it is directed to our bones and not our hearts. Many of the beneficial functions of vitamin D are only fully realized when both vitamin D and vitamin A bind to their respective nuclear receptors in the cell and form a complex that regulates the expression of certain genes. Excessive levels of vitamin D can disrupt this synergistic relationship.[192] In addition, vitamin A

---

191 Thomas F. Ferris, et al., "Renal Potassium-Wasting Induced by Vitamin D," *The Journal of Clinical Investigation* 41, no. 4 (1962): 710–716.

192 First, by competing for shared nuclear receptors and potentially disrupting vitamin A's role in gene expression, and second, by raising calcium levels to a degree that requires additional vitamin A to help manage calcium homeostasis in the blood.

is critical for assisting copper in regulating iron, a process that excess vitamin D can interfere with.

Likely for these reasons, a significant 2013 study found no clinical benefit for vitamin D stores above 21 ng/mL, a level well below the reference range on most standard blood panels.[193] More troubling, further research suggests that high levels of storage D, or levels that would be considered optimal by medical authorities, actually increase the risk of all-cause mortality, as well as the risk of heart disease and cancer.[194]

God's design is clear in this case: vitamin D should come primarily from sunlight, and secondarily from whole food sources where it is balanced by vitamin A and other cofactors.

Supplemental Calcium

Calcium is essential, but calcium supplements are not. As people age, especially women, bone density often declines, leading many to turn to calcium pills. Morley Robbins calls this the "simple lie." The "complex truth" is that this bone loss is rarely due to a lack of calcium, but rather to an excess of unbound iron that destroys bone-building cells.[195]

Research clearly shows that while supplemental calcium increases calcium levels, it doesn't reduce bone loss or improve bone remodeling.[196] Instead, excess calcium from supplements often calcifies soft tissues, including arteries, which increases the risk of heart disease.

---

193 Muhammad Amer and Rehan Qayyum, "Relationship Between 25-Hydroxyvitamin D and All-Cause and Cardiovascular Disease Mortality," *The American Journal of Medicine* 126, no. 6 (June 2013): 509–14.

194 Christine L. Taylor et al., "Questions About Vitamin D for Primary Care Practice: Input From an NIH Conference," *The American Journal of Medicine* 128, no. 11 (November 2015): 1167–70.

195 Robbins, *Cu-RE Your Fatigue.*

196 Ian R. Reid, Sarah M. Bristow, and Mark J. Bolland, "Calcium Supplements: Benefits and Risks," *Journal of Internal Medicine* 278, no. 4 (2015): 354–368.

For this reason, one review found calcium supplementation significantly increased the risk of heart attack.[197]

Robbins points out that the human diet has historically maintained a 1:1 ratio of calcium to magnesium, a balance found in whole foods such as seeds and nuts. Today, calcium intake has surged—largely from dairy products—while magnesium intake has declined, creating a 5:1 imbalance in favor of calcium.[198] This shift poses a serious problem because magnesium is essential for activating calcium's bone-building benefits, and excess calcium inhibits magnesium absorption.[199]

The bottom line is that calcium is abundant in whole foods, and when consumed in balance with magnesium and other important vitamins and minerals, it supports healthy bones. Supplements, however, have not been shown to provide any benefit and may cause harm.

Supplemental Zinc

Zinc, while essential for health, can have harmful effects when taken as a supplement (a recurring theme). In this case, excess zinc disrupts copper and iron metabolism, impairing clean energy production and potentially increasing oxidative stress.

Food-based zinc enters the system slowly and in a balanced form. Supplemental zinc, on the other hand, floods the system quickly, prompting the liver to produce metallothionein, a metal-binding protein that protects against metal toxicity (from zinc, cadmium, and mercury, for example). The problem is that metallothionein has an affinity for copper that is 1,000 times stronger than for zinc. As a result, excess zinc indirectly sequesters copper, especially in the liver, where it's most needed for essential metabolic processes.

---

197 Mark J. Bolland, "Calcium Supplements and Cardiovascular Risk: 5 Years On," *Therapeutic Advances in Drug Safety* 9, no. 8 (2018): 259–268, https://doi.org/10.1177/2042098618781515.

198 Andrea Rosanoff, Connie M. Weaver, and Richard K. Rude, "Suboptimal Magnesium Status in the United States: Are the Health Consequences Underestimated?" *Nutrition Reviews* 70, no. 3 (2012): 153–164, https://doi.org/10.1111/j.1753-4887.2011.00465.x.

199 Robbins, *Cu-RE Your Fatigue.*

To add insult to injury, zinc inhibits the activity of ceruloplasmin, the bioactive form of copper that is critical for converting ferrous iron (Fe^{2+}) to its ferric form (Fe^{3+}). This conversion is essential for proper iron transport and storage, and without it, iron remains in a reactive state that promotes oxidative stress.

The combined effect of copper sequestration and ceruloplasmin inhibition delivers a "one–two punch" to the body's clean energy production. While zinc is indeed an important mineral, it's best obtained from whole foods, where it's naturally balanced with other essential cofactors.

Moving Forward by Turning Backward

In conclusion, simply fixing our relationship with carbohydrates, ditching ultra-processed oils, minimizing the consumption of harmful pesticides, and re-evaluating how the commonly recommended supplements and enriched foods we consume can negatively impact our critical vitamin and mineral balances is the first and perhaps greatest step toward a diet that promotes strength for life and minimizes the potential for metabolic dysfunction. However, given the abundance of ultra-processed and chemically altered "food-like" substances in our daily lives, removing them from our pantries may leave some of us apprehensively wondering, "What's left that I *can* eat?"

Thankfully, we are not left empty-handed. God has provided what we might call the five "Pillars of the Plate"—the essential nutrients and food sources that we should prioritize in order to reclaim or optimize health. The task of the next chapter will be to explore these pillars in depth, revealing a more inclusive and satisfying approach to nutrition than many modern dietary guidelines would suggest is possible—one that is more reminiscent of God's abundant provision than any frying pan of reconstituted machine lubricant could ever hope to offer.

Do "Unclean" Foods Harm Metabolic Health?

It's important to note that biblically "unclean" foods are absent from this collection of top metabolic disruptors. As discussed in Chapter Two, there's no reason to believe that health was the basis for the food distinctions under the Law of Moses. Still, some have suggested that these ancient distinctions might nevertheless overlap with health risks, as the symbolic categories of the law may also have biological relevance. Do the now-obsolete categories of clean and unclean foods map neatly onto human health? The short answer is no.

Consider camels and cows. The former was once deemed detestable, the latter "clean." Yet the meat of both animals (each a ruminant) is nearly identical from a nutritional standpoint. Likewise, while pork was prohibited and chicken permitted, their modern health impacts have far more to do with how they're raised and fed than with any biblical designation. (We'll revisit this in Chapter Ten when discussing the metabolic differences between ruminants and single-stomached animals.)

Weston A. Price's early twentieth-century research offers a fascinating example of cultures that never knew the Mosaic dietary laws, eating instead according to the accumulated health wisdom of their ancestors. He observed that many traditional peoples thrived on diets rich in foods considered "unclean" by Mosaic standards. The isolated Gaelics ate lobster; the Eskimos, seal oil and whale skin; the Melanesians, wild pigs and coconut crabs. Yet these groups exhibited remarkable vitality— broad faces, strong teeth, and near-immunity to degenerative disease. It was only when they began trading with Westerners and consuming refined flours, canned goods, and sweets that their health declined rapidly, marked by crooked teeth, weakened immunity, and other modern ailments. The true target of this chapter is not traditional fare, clean or unclean, but the Western diet that displaced it.

8

Pillars of the Plate (Foundational Foods for Metabolic Health)

"The eyes of all look to you, and you give them
their food in due season. You open your hand;
you satisfy the desire of every living thing."

— PSALM 145:15–16

R educing or eliminating the main culprits of metabolic dysfunction is a crucial first step in cultivating a healthier relationship with food. The next step is to replace these man-made staples of the modern diet with the foods God created for our well-being—our "daily bread," so to speak.

The "Pillars of the Plate" are not an exhaustive list of acceptable foods, but rather serve as essential focal points for building a diet that promotes optimal health—or strength for life, as we've defined it. Centering our diet around these five key elements—quality protein, natural fats, fiber, fermented foods, and specifically targeted micronutrients—not only aligns with ancestral eating patterns, but also reflects the Logos of creation, providing our cells with the building blocks, energy, and information that they expect.

Quality Protein

Proteins are the foundational building blocks of the body. Muscle tissue, hormones, neurotransmitters, enzymes, and just about everything else that makes the body work rely on them. However, unlike fat and carbohydrates, the body has no storage reservoir for protein. It must consistently come from food or, alternatively, from muscle breakdown; there's no other option. This dependence underscores the importance of dietary protein in God's design for human flourishing.

The "protein leverage hypothesis" offers a scientific explanation for our apparent natural preference for protein, suggesting that human appetite is regulated primarily to achieve a target level of protein intake. According to this theory, protein is so vital that we're wired to keep eating until we've consumed enough of it. This would certainly explain why protein has a greater effect on suppressing ghrelin (the hunger hormone) and increasing satiety hormones than other macronutrients.

A growing body of evidence supports the need to prioritize protein, making quality protein the first of the five Pillars of the Plate.

What Defines a "Quality" Protein?

To understand what is meant by the term "quality protein," we must first explore how dietary protein functions.

It's important to remember that the body doesn't make proteins directly from protein; instead, it breaks down dietary protein into smaller units called amino acids. These amino acids enter the bloodstream and travel to cells, where they are arranged into specific functional sequences, much like a writer arranges letters into words and sentences. But while letters are free and limited only by the writer's willingness to press a key on the keyboard, imagine if some letters had a cap on their use.

For example, imagine trying to write a book about Dr. Seuss's character Zizzer-Zazzer-Zuzz using only the letters found in the book *Green Eggs and Ham*. While the total number of letters might be sufficient, the Zs would quickly be exhausted, making the task impossible. Cells operate under a similar cap—they can only build new proteins if all the necessary amino acids are present. If even a single amino acid is missing, the protein won't be made. Therefore, getting all the necessary amino acids into the cell in the right proportions is the key to making all the functional proteins the body needs to build and repair itself.

It's important to understand that amino acids share the same basic backbone of carbon, hydrogen, and oxygen found in fats and carbohydrates, yet they carry an extra component—nitrogen (and, for a few, sulfur). That added nitrogen is what allows amino acids to link into the complex three-dimensional structures we call proteins. Because their carbon-hydrogen-oxygen skeleton looks so familiar to the cell, amino acids can be routed down two very different paths: they can be re-assembled into new proteins or stripped of their nitrogen and burned for energy, with the liberated nitrogen converted to urea and excreted by the kidneys. Measuring that urea tells us how much of each pathway is in use.

Whether amino acids are used for construction or energy depends largely on the composition of the amino acid profile. Protein sources with the right balance of amino acids are more likely to be used for building. Essential amino acids (EAAs)—those that the body cannot synthesize and must obtain from food—are particularly critical, and are more likely to be utilized than the non-essential amino acids. They are like the Zs in the Dr. Suess analogy—the most highly prized letters.

Protein sources that contain all nine EAAs are considered "complete" and are highly valued for their efficiency in protein synthesis. But even among the EAAs, some amino acids are more important than others. For example, our cells have sensors that specifically look for leucine, an EAA that can single-handedly stimulate muscle protein synthesis.

With this understanding in mind, we can conclude that a protein source has two important characteristics that determine its quality:

1. *absorption*—how efficiently its amino acids reach the bloodstream; and

2. *utilization*—how effectively those amino acids are used to build proteins rather than being converted to energy.

Animal-based proteins generally excel in both categories, offering all essential amino acids in ratios that are highly useful to the human body. Whole eggs are the best source,[200] followed closely by dairy and meat products.[201] While plant-based proteins, such as quinoa, lentils, chickpeas, and pumpkin seeds, can also provide a notable amount of protein, they tend to be less easily absorbed and lack a complete amino acid profile on their own.[202] We'll discuss these differences in more detail in Chapter Ten.

How Much Protein Do We Need?

While determining the *quality* of a protein source is relatively straightforward, determining the optimal *quantity* is far more controversial.

The recommended daily allowance (RDA) for protein is just 0.8 grams per kilogram of body weight—a measly 65 grams for a 180-pound man and only 42 grams for a 115-pound woman. This recommendation hasn't changed since the 1980s and was originally based on nitrogen balance studies conducted primarily on healthy young men, a highly flawed approach that has been extensively criticized for underestimating actual protein needs.[203] It also incorrectly assumes that all protein is of

---

200 Contrary to popular belief, egg whites alone aren't nearly as potent a protein source as the whole thing, yolk and all. One study published in the *Journal of Nutrition* found that consuming whole eggs rather than just the whites leads to greater muscle protein synthesis following exercise. The yolk adds phospholipids, fats, vitamins, minerals, and essential amino acids that combine to make the protein more highly absorbed and utilized.

201 Insaf Berrazaga et al., "The Role of the Anabolic Properties of Plant- versus Animal-Based Protein Sources in Supporting Muscle Mass Maintenance: A Critical Review," *Nutrients* 11, no. 8 (August 7, 2019): 1825.

202 Ibid.

203 Mary Weiler, Steven R. Hertzler, and Svyatoslav Dvoretskiy. 2023. "Is It Time to Reconsider the US Recommendations for Dietary Protein and Amino Acid Intake?" *Nutrients* 15, no. 4: 838.

equal quality, while we know now that what matters isn't necessarily the weight of protein consumed, but rather the amount of critical amino acids that make it to the cells. At best, the RDA prevents severe deficiencies but falls short of supporting optimal health, especially for older adults, active individuals, pregnant or nursing women, and those recovering from illness or injury.

If our diets are to produce optimal strength for life, it's not enough to avoid severe protein deficiency. Instead, given that skeletal muscle is arguably the most important metabolic organ, our protein intake should be directed toward optimizing muscle maintenance and growth.

Dr. Gabrielle Lyon recommends consuming 1 gram of quality protein per pound of "ideal body weight" to promote muscle health, regardless of age or gender. According to Lyon, ideal body weight doesn't necessarily refer to a person's current weight, but rather a theoretical weight that is consistent with optimal body composition and health. For example, a man who weighs 180 pounds but is aiming for a leaner, healthier, "ideal" weight of 175 pounds would aim to consume 175 grams of protein per day. Similarly, a woman who weighs 115 pounds and wants to gain 10 pounds of muscle mass might aim for 125 grams of protein per day. This is nearly three times the standard RDA!

Lyon's recommendation is certainly on the high end of the protein intake spectrum and may only be necessary for those with higher protein needs. An alternative, potentially more practical, guideline is to consume about 1 gram of quality protein per pound of *lean* body weight. Unlike the concept of ideal body weight, which represents a goal, lean body weight is a measurable figure calculated by subtracting body fat from total body weight. For example, a 180-pound man with 20 percent body fat has a lean body weight of 144 pounds and would aim for 144 grams of protein daily—a recommendation closer to twice the RDA.

Both rules of thumb emphasize eating to support muscle protein synthesis, but in doing so, they naturally promote some other metabolic benefits.

For example, because protein is highly satiating, it helps to regulate portion size and discourage overeating. As most of us have experienced, even the best dieting intentions tend to be unsuccessful to the extent that they pit willpower against bodily cues, as our body chemistry often wins. By prioritizing protein, we promote the proper balance between our needs and our desires, helping to properly order our will according to our body's true needs.

Protein also enhances thermogenesis because it requires more energy to digest, absorb, and metabolize than other macronutrients. This increased energy expenditure improves body composition and promotes metabolic balance.

Given its many metabolic benefits, optimizing protein intake should be a top dietary priority, making quality protein the cornerstone of the five Pillars of the Plate.

Natural Fats

"My soul will be satisfied as with fat
and rich food, And my mouth will
praise you with joyful lips."

— PSALM 63:5

"On this mountain the Lord of hosts will
make for all peoples a feast of rich food,
a feast of well-aged wine, of rich food full
of marrow, of aged wine well refined."

— ISAIAH 25:6

Those who have been following standard nutritional advice since the 1950s may be unfamiliar with the taste of bone marrow and miss the intended effect of Isaiah's prophecy describing the richness of the heavenly banquet. Could Isaiah have been mistaken? Surely, we won't be eating "artery-clogging" saturated fat in heaven!

We've already discussed the dangers of ultra-processed oils, noting that these toxic PUFAs were introduced into the modern diet to replace traditional fats. But if quality protein is to be the first priority in our diet, then we should appeal to the Logos of creation, which dictates that quality protein sources almost always come with fat.

Think about it—meat, eggs, dairy products, nuts, and seeds are rich in both protein and fat. These natural fats should not be feared, but rather welcomed as essential components of a healthy diet. They've sustained humanity for millennia, providing clean energy, reducing inflammation, restoring hormonal balance, and preventing metabolic dysfunction.

However, to understand how traditional fats fit into a biblical nutritional paradigm, we must revisit the historical missteps that led to their demonization.

The Low-Fat Fiasco

Heart disease was once a rare problem, and cardiology was barely recognized as a field, but President Eisenhower's first heart attack in 1955 brought national attention to the issue and spurred increased funding and research into its prevention. By then, Ancel Keys, a charismatic and influential physiologist, had developed a theory that dietary fat—particularly saturated fat—was the main driver of heart disease. His reasoning was straightforward: saturated fat raises cholesterol, elevated cholesterol clogs arteries, and clogged arteries lead to heart attacks.

In 1957, Keys presented his now famous "Six Countries Study" at a WHO conference in Geneva, aiming to demonstrate the link between saturated fat intake and heart disease. His graph showed a clear correlation between saturated fat consumption and heart disease rates in Finland, Greece, Italy, Japan, the Netherlands, and the United States. Japan, with its low-fat diet, had minimal heart disease, while the US, with its high-fat diet, had high rates. Sure enough, the remaining four countries filled in the gaps, seemingly proving his hypothesis.[204]

But Keys's observational study faced strong criticism. His colleagues first pointed out that correlation doesn't prove causation. What if the

---

204 Ancel Keys, "Atherosclerosis: A Problem in Newer Public Health," *Journal of the Mount Sinai Hospital, New York* 20, no. 2 (1953): 118–39.

saturated fat eaters in the US were also heavy smokers? And why did Keys choose six countries when data were available for 22? Critics accused him of cherry-picking data, noting the exclusion of France, which had a notoriously fatty cuisine but low rates of heart disease.[205]

The attacks didn't stop Keys from becoming a celebrity scientist, authoring several other high-profile studies over the years, and even appearing on the cover of *Time* magazine in 1961.[206] Although controversial and heavily criticized ever since, Keys's research has permeated not only the public consciousness but also the medical, pharmaceutical, and food industries, still informing the claims of prominent health organizations such as the American Heart Association.

Yet his most rigorous study, the Minnesota Coronary Experiment (1968–1973), never made the news—largely because it was never even published. Unlike his earlier observational studies, which relied on national dietary surveys, food balance sheets, and self-reported eating habits—methods notorious for their inaccuracy and susceptibility to confounding factors—this randomized controlled trial was designed to definitively prove whether replacing saturated fat with PUFA-rich ultra-processed oils would reduce cholesterol and heart disease. The study used a tightly controlled environment, tracking thousands of patients in state mental hospitals and nursing homes, where every meal was prepared and carefully monitored to control fat intake, but the results didn't turn out as he had envisioned. Keys was horrified to find that while the ultra-processed oil group did indeed experience lower cholesterol levels, they showed no improvement in heart disease or all-cause mortality. Worse, these participants experienced a 22 percent *higher* risk of death for every 30 mg/dL reduction in cholesterol. That's right—the cholesterol-lowering oils were shown to *cause* death, not

---

205 J. Yerushalmy and H. E. Hilleboe, "Fat in the Diet and Mortality from Heart Disease: A Methodologic Note," *New York State Journal of Medicine* 57, no. 14 (1957): 2343–54.
206 "Medicine: The Fat of the Land," *TIME*, January 13, 1961.

prevent it. Keys apparently buried the study that contradicted his hypothesis for decades.[207]

Reexamining Cholesterol

Although saturated fat raises cholesterol levels, the notion that this causes clogged arteries has been thoroughly debunked. In reality, the relationship between cholesterol and heart health is far more complex than we are often led to believe.

Cholesterol, a waxy, fat-like substance, is a critical component of cell membranes and a precursor to several essential hormones. Contrary to popular belief, dietary cholesterol from sources such as eggs has minimal effect on blood cholesterol levels because it is poorly absorbed by the body. The liver produces and regulates the vast majority of cholesterol, regardless of dietary intake. However, because cholesterol is hydrophobic (not soluble in water), it cannot move freely in the bloodstream. Instead, it is encased in a protein shell called a lipoprotein, which transports cholesterol throughout the body and delivers it to where it is needed. Standard lipid panels measure these lipoproteins, focusing on two types: LDL (low-density lipoprotein) and HDL (high-density lipoprotein).

LDL is often called "bad" cholesterol because it can build up in arterial walls when there's too much of it, while HDL is called "good" because it acts like a vacuum cleaner, picking up old lipoproteins and depositing them back in the liver. But this antiquated paradigm oversimplifies the truth. While HDL is indeed very healthy, LDL doesn't necessarily deserve its reputation as a cardiovascular menace.

Research now shows that it's not LDL itself, but rather *oxidized* LDL particles that build up in the arteries and form plaques—a subtle but important distinction. What triggers this oxidation in the first place? According to a comprehensive review by James DiNicolantonio and

---

207   Christopher E. Ramsden et al., "Re-evaluation of the Traditional Diet-heart Hypothesis: Analysis of Recovered Data From Minnesota Coronary Experiment (1968-73)," *BMJ* (April 2016): i1246.

James O'Keefe, omega-6 PUFAs from ultra-processed oils, not saturated fat, are major contributors to LDL oxidation. This finding helps explain the unexpected results of the Minnesota Coronary Experiment. Their review shows that the fats from these oils accumulate inside LDL particles, where their instability makes them highly prone to oxidation, resulting in the oxidation of the entire LDL particle. Once oxidized, these LDL particles are no longer recognized by the liver and are instead managed by the immune system, leading to the formation of foam cells—a hallmark of atherogenic plaques.[208]

Another reason LDL levels alone are a poor indicator of cardiovascular risk is that standard tests assume all LDL particles are identical. In reality, LDL particles vary in size and density, each carrying a different level of risk. Large, fluffy, buoyant "Pattern A" LDL particles, which comprise the majority of LDL, are relatively harmless. By contrast, small, dense "Pattern B" LDL particles are highly predictive of heart disease. These smaller particles are more prone to oxidation, more likely to penetrate arterial walls, and tend to stay in circulation longer, increasing their potential to cause harm.[209][210]

Paradoxically, elevated levels of small, dense LDL particles are not driven by saturated fat intake. These particles often carry triglycerides, which are produced by the liver when there is an overload of sugar, particularly refined sugar and fructose. In other words, it's excessive sugar—not fat—that promotes the formation of these harmful particles. To make matters worse, the "good" HDL particles have to work harder

---

208 DiNicolantonio and O'Keefe, "Omega-6 Vegetable Oils as a Driver of Coronary Heart Disease: The Oxidized Linoleic Acid Hypothesis."

209 Remember that the liver is the internal cashier of metabolism, so when its glycogen stores are full, it takes free fatty acids (from insulin-resistant fat cells) and triglycerides converted from excess sugar (especially fructose) and packages them into special carriers called very-low-density lipoproteins (VLDL). Once these VLDLs enter the bloodstream, they tend to shrink as they shed their fats and become small, dense LDL particles. This is explained in more depth in Isabella Bonilha et al., "The Reciprocal Relationship Between LDL Metabolism and Type 2 Diabetes Mellitus," *Metabolites* 11, no. 12 (November 2021): 807.

210 Measuring the triglyceride-to-HDL ratio is the best low cost method of assessing the predominant size and density of LDL particles in the blood. The lower the ratio the better, with 1 or less being optimal and 2 or higher starting to indicate both insulin resistance and a pattern of small, dense LDL particles.

to remove the extra lipids and transport them back to the liver, quickly depleting their concentration in the blood.[211]

In short, heart disease is not a problem of high cholesterol; it's a problem of metabolic dysfunction. Cholesterol is often just an innocent bystander caught up in the mess, and only then does it play a role in heart disease.

This has been borne out in several large observational studies. For example, one study of US adults not being treated for high cholesterol found a U-shaped relationship between LDL cholesterol and all-cause mortality, with the lowest risk occurring between 110–190 mg/dL—even though conventional guidelines often recommend staying below 100 mg/dL.[212] A similar study out of Denmark found the lowest mortality at an LDL level of about 140 mg/dL, a number that might raise eyebrows among conventionally trained cardiologists.[213] In both studies, the best predictor of mortality wasn't LDL, but the triglyceride-to-HDL ratio, with a value of 1 or less being ideal.

It's worth noting that this U-shaped curve isn't exactly symmetrical: there tends to be more risk at the low end of the LDL spectrum than at the high end. Still, elevated LDL may carry some risk in these general population cohorts. However, cholesterol researcher Dave Feldman has compiled several studies showing that even people with very high LDL—upward of 300 mg/dL—don't develop arterial plaque if they're metabolically healthy. In lean individuals with low inflammation and

---

211 Most people don't understand that statins—the commonly prescribed class of drugs aimed at lowering LDL cholesterol—only lower the concentration of the harmless, "Pattern A" LDL particles, which is why they have been shown to have very little protective effect despite significant adverse side effects.

212 Salami, Joseph A., et al. "Association of Low-Density Lipoprotein Cholesterol With Risk of All-Cause and Cause-Specific Mortality in the Contemporary Era: A Large Cohort Study of United States Adults." Journal of the American Heart Association 6, no. 12 (2017): e006879. https://doi.org/10.1161/JAHA.117.006879.

213 Christian D. L. Johannesen, Anne Langsted, Bo M. Mortensen, et al., "Association Between Low-Density Lipoprotein and All-Cause and Cause-Specific Mortality in Denmark: Prospective Cohort Study," BMJ 371 (2020): m4266, https://doi.org/10.1136/bmj.m4266.

good blood-sugar control, his data show no link between LDL levels and plaque buildup.

So what about the healthiest of the healthy? A large and comprehensive longitudinal study comparing centenarians to the general population found that one of the strongest predictors of living to one hundred is, somewhat counterintuitively, high cholesterol![214]

Therefore, claiming that cholesterol causes heart disease is like saying that wood causes house fires. Yes, wood is often found at the scene of a fire—but that doesn't mean it started the blaze. In fact, wood is an essential building material, just as LDL cholesterol is vital for many purposes in the body. It is only when a fire is already burning—when the body is inflamed or oxidatively stressed—that LDL becomes damaged and contributes to arterial plaque. By targeting the actual sources of metabolic fire—largely through a diet based on God's design—we address the root causes of heart disease rather than blaming the building materials.

Embracing All Natural Fats

All natural fats—saturated, monounsaturated, and polyunsaturated—are essential to a balanced diet. Incorporating traditional yet often stigmatized fats, such as cream, lard, and tallow, alongside universally praised options like avocado and coconut oil, not only promotes nutritional balance but also enhances the richness and flavor of our meals.

In this context, grass-fed butter emerges as a healthy food rather than a dietary threat, providing stable saturated fats, fat-soluble vitamins, and beneficial compounds such as butyrate and conjugated linoleic acid (CLA). Similarly, grass-fed beef tallow has long been a culinary favorite. Compared to flavorless and toxic oils, tallow is both incredibly nutrient

---

214 Shunsuke Murata et al., "Blood Biomarker Profiles and Exceptional Longevity: Comparison of Centenarians and Non-Centenarians in a 35-Year Follow-Up of the Swedish AMORIS Cohort," *GeroScience*, 2024.

dense and has a high smoke point, making it a stable and heart healthy option for sautéing and high-heat cooking.

On the plant-based side, extra virgin coconut oil is a fantastic source of a variety of fats. Among these, its medium-chain triglycerides (MCTs) stand out for their rapid absorption and ability to be converted by the liver into ketones, which serve as an important source of energy and a signaling molecule that improves mitochondrial function.[215] Olive oil (first cold pressed, extra virgin) is another health-affirming fat source that provides a host of antioxidants and polyphenols and acts as a potent anti-inflammatory. While it has a higher content of PUFAs than these other sources, they are preserved intact through delicate extraction methods and are protected by the other healthy compounds in the oil.

Whether it's these, ghee, avocado oil, or any other natural source of fat that hasn't been mangled beyond recognition, the point is the same: the fats that appeal to the logic of God's created order are indeed very good.

Are "Health Foods" Expensive?

There is a pervasive idea that healthy eating is prohibitively expensive. Locally sourced raw milk often costs twice as much as mass-produced alternatives, sprouted breads can cost three times as much as generic white breads, and pasture-raised eggs with butter can seem extravagant compared to instant oatmeal. It's easy to see why these foods might be dismissed as luxuries, seemingly at odds with the Christian call to financial stewardship.

Simply put, this perception is in dire need of a reality check. For most of human history, securing food consumed the better part of one's time and resources. Today, even the finest steak dinner represents only a small fraction of the average person's labor. While it's true that quality food is more expensive than its mass-produced counterparts, it's still far cheaper than at any other time in human history, when food was often a household's largest expense.

---

215 We'll discuss these in more depth in Chapter Nine.

The belief that real food is too expensive is driven in part by the artificially low prices of ultra-processed, nutrient-deficient food-like substances that are kept cheap by heavy subsidies. These items appear affordable at the checkout counter, but their hidden costs—chronic disease, mounting medical bills, lost productivity, and disastrous environmental outcomes—don't show up on the receipt.

Investing in high-quality, nutrient-dense food is an investment in long-term health and well-being. Don't be fooled by the superficial affordability of ultra-processed foods; the true cost is far greater.

Fiber

Throughout history, the curious tale of Esau trading his birthright for a bowl of lentil soup has puzzled many. Was it sheer hunger, or was there more to this biblical story?

Upon closer inspection, Esau wasn't entirely misguided in his craving—though certainly reckless in his timing. After all, lentils are rich in one thing we can easily overlook: fiber. Was it worth its weight in birthrights? Perhaps not. But while the typical Western diet is loaded with refined grains, industrial fats, and toxins, we have largely lost the simple wisdom that Esau's appetite hints at—that food rich in natural fiber can powerfully support digestion and metabolic health.

The average American consumes about half of the recommended 25–30 grams of fiber per day, a benchmark that nearly 95 percent of the population fails to meet. Yet even this recommendation can be overly simplistic, since not all fiber is the same, and not everyone benefits equally from it.[216]

---

216 For some people, such as those with irritable bowel syndrome (IBS), small intestinal bacterial overgrowth (SIBO), or certain inflammatory gut conditions, high fiber foods can aggravate symptoms and may need to be limited. Furthermore, people well-adapted to very low carbohydrate diets, such as the carnivore diet, have bowels that function via bile acids, fat metabolism, and microbial adaptation, not bulk fiber.

Fiber comes in two forms—soluble and insoluble—each with distinct benefits for many people.

Soluble Fiber. Soluble fiber dissolves in water to form a gel-like substance and can be fermented by gut bacteria. Found in foods like oats, legumes (beans, lentils, peas), nuts, seeds, some fruits (like apples and blueberries), and vegetables, soluble fiber can aid digestion, soften stool, and support bowel regularity. Metabolically, it can slow digestion, promote satiety, and reduce post-meal blood sugar spikes.

Within this category, *prebiotic* fibers stand out for feeding beneficial gut bacteria and promoting the production of SCFAs. Inulin, for instance, found in Jerusalem artichokes, chicory, garlic, onions, leeks, and asparagus, stimulates butyrate production. Psyllium husk and soaked basil seeds are other potent, accessible sources of prebiotic fiber.

Insoluble Fiber. Insoluble fiber, which does not dissolve in water and passes through the digestive system largely intact, promotes regularity by speeding the movement of material through the intestines and adding bulk to stool. This type of fiber is found primarily in whole grains, nuts, seeds, and the skins or structural elements of many fruits and vegetables.

Unfortunately, modern food processing often strips away fiber to extend shelf life. This is why a diet abundant in whole fruits, vegetables, nuts, seeds, and certain grains tends to support better digestion and metabolic balance. While fiber is not strictly essential for health, many people find that consuming a variety of natural, fiber-rich foods enhances gut function and overall well-being. In a world dominated by refined, low-fiber fare, such foods represent one of the simplest, most restorative choices we can make for lifelong health.

Fermented Foods

Unfortunately, while fiber consumption offers several benefits, it can't single-handedly ensure optimal gut health.

Research conducted at Stanford University has shown that while a high-fiber diet supports the proliferation of some gut bacteria, it doesn't necessarily increase microbial diversity. Study participants who significantly increased their fiber intake without increasing their consumption of fermented foods experienced higher densities of some microbes, but not much else. Conversely, participants who maintained their usual fiber intake but significantly increased their consumption of fermented foods, such as yogurt, kefir, kombucha, sauerkraut, and kimchi, experienced both a notable increase in microbial diversity and a corresponding decrease in inflammatory markers.[217] These findings underscore the importance of combining high-fiber foods with fermented products to cultivate a gut microbiome that is both robust and diverse.

Humans have relied on this Pillar of the Plate for thousands of years. Herodotus, the esteemed fifth-century BC historian, noted, "Egyptians set aside their dough until it decayed, and observed with pleasure the process that took place."[218] While fermentation likely gained popularity for its role in preserving food and enhancing flavor, its benefits extend far beyond these practical advantages. The microorganisms involved in fermentation—bacteria, yeasts, and molds—act as miniature nutrient factories, synthesizing and releasing nutrients otherwise unavailable to humans. This process enhances the nutritional value of food, neutralizes toxins, and fosters a thriving gut ecosystem.

For example, yeast-driven fermentation in bread-making significantly improves the nutritional profile of wheat-based products. Wheat and other seeds contain anti-nutrient proteins called phytates that bind essential minerals such as calcium, magnesium, and zinc. While these phytates are essential for plant development, they interfere with mineral absorption during the human digestive process. Enzymes in yeast, however, break down phytates, freeing these minerals for absorption. This microbial intervention not only improves the taste and texture of food, but also its nutritional value, highlighting the

---

217   Hannah C. Wastyk et al., "Gut-Microbiota-Targeted Diets Modulate Human Immune Status," *Cell* 184, no. 16 (August 2021): 4137-4153.e14.

218   As cited in H. E. Jacob, *Six Thousand Years of Bread* (New York: Skyhorse Publishing Inc., 2007).

indispensable role of fermentation in human nutrition.[219] Without these processes, many nutrients would remain trapped within food structures, passing through the digestive system without delivering their full health benefits.

Similarly, while often marketed as superior alternatives to dairy and meat, most mass-produced soy milk, tofu, and other soy products are anything but health foods. Ancient cultures, perhaps through trial and error, recognized the limitations of raw soybeans, which contain several anti-nutrient compounds. But when these beans are rinsed, soaked, and fermented, their nutrients are released and the toxins are neutralized, creating the traditional tofu, natto, miso, and other cultured soy products that are an integral part of some cuisines.

For example, while soybeans are rich in protein, their protein quality is compromised by trypsin inhibitors that hinder digestion. Fermentation not only breaks down soy protein into more digestible amino acids but also significantly reduces the presence of these anti-nutrients, making it more bioavailable. In addition, fermentation enriches soy products with essential nutrients such as B vitamins and vitamin K_2, thanks to the beneficial microbes involved.

Raw soybeans are also loaded with toxins called goitrogens and phytoestrogens. Goitrogens disrupt thyroid function by blocking iodine absorption, while phytoestrogens mimic or interfere with the body's estrogen, potentially impacting fertility and thyroid health. Concerns have been raised about raw soy's association with thyroid disorders, including both hypo- and hyperthyroidism, as well as thyroid cancer and fertility issues. Fortunately, while cooking only partially reduces the bioavailability of these compounds, fermentation largely neutralizes them, significantly reducing the risks associated with raw soy consumption.

Beyond neutralizing anti-nutrients and improving the nutritional profile of foods, fermented and cultured foods are often touted as "living

---

219   Kenneth F. *Kiple* and Kriemhild Coneè Ornelas, eds., *The Cambridge World History of Food*, vol. 2 (Cambridge: Cambridge University Press, 2000), 1473, as cited in Cate Shanahan, *Deep Nutrition: Why Your Genes Need Traditional Food* (New York: Flatiron Books, 2017).

foods" due to their "live and active" bacterial cultures. However, many of these bacteria are no longer alive by the time the food is consumed or fail to survive digestion. Surprisingly, this doesn't diminish their value. The Stanford study revealed that much of the microbial diversity attributed to a high-fermented diet didn't come directly from the bacteria in the fermented foods themselves. This suggests that the health benefits of fermented foods extend beyond the provision of live bacteria.

The primary benefits of fermented foods, somewhat counterintuitively, may come primarily from their dead bacteria and the metabolic byproducts they produced while alive. These by-products, including *intermediate* SCFAs, are critical for the maintenance of various species of intestinal bacteria. For example, lactofermentation produces lactic acid, which contributes to tangy flavors and lowers pH for preservation. But while lactic acid has no direct health benefit, it serves as a vital food source for many species of gut bacteria that produce butyrate and other beneficial SCFAs.

Even dead bacteria play an important signaling role in gut health. A recent study comparing the effects of feeding mice either live or dead Akkermansia found that both forms provided unique benefits. While live bacteria helped maintain gut homeostasis and influenced genes related to metabolism and immune function, dead bacteria were more effective in strengthening the gut barrier, reducing inflammation, and preventing leakage.[220] While delicacies such as aged wines, champagnes, cheeses, and vinegars are devoid of live bacteria, they remain rich in the nutrients these creatures produced while alive. Just as important, these deceased microbes make significant contributions from the grave, providing spare parts and a valuable signaling role that stimulates health in ways that science is only beginning to unravel.

The marvel of our ancestors' ability to harness the power of invisible microbes was considered nothing short of miraculous by the ancients, who attributed the sophisticated arts of wine and bread making to divine intervention rather than human ingenuity. This reverence

---

220 Fatemeh Ashrafian et al., "Comparative Effects of Alive and Pasteurized *Akkermansia muciniphila* on Normal Diet-Fed Mice," *Scientific Reports* 11, no. 1 (September 2021) (as cited in Gundry, *Gut Check*).

underscores a deep respect for the natural processes that were beyond their complete understanding and honors these practices as sacred gifts rather than mere culinary techniques.

Today, despite our advanced understanding of microbes and their myriad benefits, modern society has turned to sterile, commercially produced foods, distancing us from the rich traditions that characterized ancestral diets. Rediscovering traditional food preparation methods—fermenting, soaking, and sprouting—can provide tremendous health benefits by improving the nutritional profile and digestibility of foods while reintroducing beneficial microbes to our gut flora. In doing so, we would not only pay homage to the ancient wisdom that has sustained human health for millennia, but also leverage it to combat the sterile and sometimes nutritionally diminished state of much modern fare.

A growing movement is celebrating fermented foods like yogurt, kefir, sauerkraut, and kimchi for their complex flavors, probiotic potential, and role in supporting a healthy microbiome. This may be a massive shift for those who believe their modern, sterile diet is normal. But for previous generations, our dead food would have been anything but.

As we move forward scientifically, we are confirming that there is much to be gained by looking backward and honoring the wisdom of our ancestors by weaving the art and science of fermentation and traditional food preparation back into the fabric of our daily lives, even if it takes a bit of open-mindedness or perhaps culinary courage!

Mind Your Micros

It's easy to get caught up in the pursuit of optimal macronutrient ratios, leading many to "count their macros" in an effort to balance carbohydrates, fats, and proteins. While this approach may have merit for some people on precisely controlled diets, it often shifts the focus away from a more important aspect of nutrition—micronutrients. If food is a pharmacy, then vitamins and minerals are its most potent medicines.

As Casey Means wisely notes, "Bites are opportunities, and you don't want to waste any. You want every bite you take to communicate with your cells about what you expect them to do."[221] Providing the body with a rich supply of essential vitamins and minerals ensures that each meal sends the right message to our cells in a language that they can understand.

But while all essential micronutrients play crucial roles in health, certain ones merit special attention as foundational pillars of a health-focused nutrition plan, either because they are particularly deficient in the modern diet or because they are uniquely effective in countering the metabolic assaults of modern life.

Supplements: Expensive Pee or a Nutritional Pillar?

Some critics dismiss supplements as merely producing "expensive pee," while others take them religiously. How do they fit into a Christian paradigm for nutrition?

We should begin by asking, "Are dietary supplements part of God's plan for human flourishing?" Given that dietary supplements have only become popular in the last century, the answer is likely "no." Many reasonably argue that if God intended us to have isolated vitamins and minerals, He would have made them grow out of the ground.

However, it's crucial to consider the counterpoint: the modern world presents unprecedented challenges to our health—constant blue light, chronic stressors, forever chemicals, depleted soils, microplastics, and polluted air and water, just for starters. In the context of unprecedented and sometimes unavoidable assaults, supplemental nutrients in the form of pills and powders may be a valuable, health-promoting tool, but with some important caveats:

---

221 Casey and Calley Means, *Good Energy*.

It's Hard to Out-Supplement an Unhealthy Lifestyle. Stewarding health should start with the foundation of a proper diet, regular exercise, adequate sleep, and exposure to sunlight. No supplement can undo the effects of an unhealthy lifestyle.

The Source Matters. Is it derived from whole foods? Minimally processed? Tested for purity and potency? These are important factors to consider.

Supplements Should Be Specific and Purposeful. Supplements should be selected with specific deficiencies or desired outcomes in mind. Most multivitamins and synthetic, broad-spectrum supplements are laden with the problematic micronutrients we discussed in the last chapter.

Vitamin C Complex

We've discussed both the shortcomings and potential dangers of supplementing with ascorbic acid, a synthetic analog of vitamin C, but enzymatically active, whole food vitamin C complex is a different story.

Naturally occurring vitamin C is critical for the adrenal glands, which synthesize cortisol and epinephrine to help the body cope with stress. Tyrosinase, the copper-containing enzyme at the heart of the vitamin C complex, acts as an adrenal activator, helping to fight adrenal fatigue.

Real vitamin C also enhances the function of lymphocytes, a type of white blood cell that is central to the immune response. Again, tyrosinase is largely responsible for this effect, strengthening the body's defenses against pathogens and infections.

Finally, vitamin C is essential for collagen synthesis. Collagen, the most abundant protein in the body, provides structural integrity to connective tissue, skin, bones, and teeth. Without sufficient vitamin C, the body's ability to repair tissue, heal wounds, and maintain healthy joints and skin is severely compromised.

The best whole food sources of vitamin C include citrus fruits (e.g., oranges, guavas, papayas), kiwis, strawberries, and raw vegetables such as bell peppers and broccoli. However, because vitamin C can degrade during shipping, supplementation may help fill the gap for those with limited access to fresh, local produce. If choosing to supplement, aim for 300–500 mg from potent food-based sources such as acerola cherries, camu camu berries, and rose hips.

Magnesium

Magnesium is essential for metabolic health, supporting approximately 80 percent of our metabolic processes. But while thousands of studies attest to its benefits, its importance as a dietary priority can be justified by three key points:

Energy Production. Without adequate magnesium, the body simply cannot produce bioavailable energy. Not only is magnesium necessary for glycolysis and key steps in the Krebs cycle, but it's also needed to stabilize every molecule of ATP. Considering that we make our body weight in ATP every day, the importance of these functions cannot be underestimated.

Combatting Stress. All forms of stress—oxidative, physical, mental, and emotional—deplete magnesium stores. Morley Robbins describes the rate at which this happens as the "magnesium burn rate." The constant stress of modern life increases this rate, leaving many people deficient and less able to cope with daily challenges.

Soil Depletion. The third observation is that our mineral-depleted soil has reduced the magnesium content of our food just when we need it most. [222]

For these reasons, aiming for 3–5 milligrams of elemental magnesium per pound of body weight per day is crucial. [223] Foods like pumpkin seeds, dark leafy greens, nuts, seeds, dark chocolate, and

---

222 A 2003 study by David Thomas, published in the journal *Nutrition and Health*, compared the mineral content of foods available in 1940 and 1991, finding that magnesium dropped 16–24 percent in our fruits and vegetables and 10 percent in meat. The copper availability in our vegetables saw the largest decline—a whopping 76 percent.

223 This recommended amount was established by Mildred Seelig, one of the pioneering magnesium researchers.

legumes are a great start, but supplementation may be necessary to address deficiencies.

Not all magnesium supplements, however, are equally effective. For example, magnesium oxide is inorganic and poorly absorbed by the body, while magnesium citrate offers only marginally better absorption. In contrast, magnesium glycinate and malate are highly bioavailable and come with additional health benefits.[224]

Electrolytes

Electrolytes are essential minerals that carry an electrical charge, enabling critical bodily functions such as hydration, nerve signaling, muscle contraction, and pH balance. Along with magnesium, the key electrolytes—sodium and potassium—must remain in proper balance to maintain homeostasis.

These two minerals play key roles in regulating the movement of water in and out of cells, ensuring that they neither shrivel from dehydration nor burst from excess fluid. Potassium draws water into cells, while sodium pulls water into the bloodstream, creating a dynamic balance crucial for cellular health.

Whole fruits and vegetables, such as bananas, avocados, potatoes, and beans, are rich in potassium. Meanwhile, sodium is best obtained from unrefined sea salt and mineral-rich broths. Supplementation may be necessary for athletes, those under chronic stress, or those on low-carb diets, as these conditions accelerate the "electrolyte burn rate," similar to the magnesium burn rate.

Sodium: A Misunderstood Mineral

In 2 Kings 2:21, when Jericho's water was causing death and miscarriages, Elisha healed it by sprinkling salt into the spring. This act of cleansing

---

224 Glycine, a vital precursor to glutathione (an important antioxidant), is the most important non-essential amino acid in the body. Malic acid is used in the Krebs cycle, which is why magnesium malate is known to be energizing and aid in preventing muscle soreness.

underscores the symbolic power of salt in Scripture—a mineral associated with preservation, purification, and covenant faithfulness. In ancient Rome, salt was so valuable that it was used as payment for soldiers, giving rise to the phrase, "worth your salt." Recognizing its enduring significance, Jesus called His followers "the salt of the earth" (Matt. 5:13), a call to season the world with flavor, preservation, and righteousness.

Today, however, salt has been vilified as both an unnecessary indulgence and a health menace. The widely promoted "salt–blood pressure hypothesis" suggests that sodium raises blood pressure by causing the body to retain excess water, leading to the widely recommended daily limit of just 2.3 grams. The truth, however, is far more nuanced. For most people, the kidneys efficiently regulate sodium levels, and it's much easier for them to excrete excess salt than to reabsorb it when levels are too low. Only about 25 percent of people—primarily those with kidney damage—are truly salt-sensitive. Not surprisingly, the real cause of both salt-sensitivity and hypertension is normally metabolic dysfunction, particularly insulin resistance, which not only raises blood pressure but also contributes to kidney damage.

Recent studies have called the war on salt into question. A 2011 study in *JAMA* found that consuming less than 3 grams of sodium daily—in line with current guidelines—increased cardiovascular risk. In contrast, those who consumed 4 to 6 grams daily—roughly double to triple the RDA—had the lowest risk of death.[225] A 2014 meta-analysis confirmed this U-shaped relationship between sodium intake and health outcomes,

---

225 K. Stolarz-Skrzypek et al., "Fatal and Nonfatal Outcomes, Incidence of Hypertension, and Blood Pressure Changes in Relation to Urinary Sodium Excretion," *JAMA* 305, no. 17 (2011): 1777–85.

finding that both too little and too much sodium increase health risks,[226] although the dangers of too little salt are far greater.[227]

The bottom line? Salt is essential, not an enemy. Most people naturally consume 3 to 6 grams per day, guided by taste, which is optimal for health.[228] However, those who switch from processed foods to whole foods may need to add more salt to their diet to reach this threshold. Just as Christians are called to season the world with righteousness, we should generously season our food with life-giving salt, embracing God's design for health and flourishing.

Retinol

In the last chapter, we explored the critical relationship between vitamins D and A, noting that they work together to regulate calcium, boost the immune system, and perform other important functions. Vitamin A also facilitates the loading of copper atoms into ceruloplasmin, the protein responsible for iron regulation. But retinol—the only bioactive form of vitamin A—is largely MIA in the Western diet.

This critical vitamin is found in foods such as liver, oily fish, cheese, butter, heavy cream, and egg yolks. With this list, it would be hard not to recognize that flavor implies nutrition! While provitamin A carotenoids—found in carrots, sweet potatoes, dark leafy greens, mangoes, and squash—can be converted to retinol, this process is far less efficient than getting it directly.

---

226 Niels Graudal, Gesche Jürgens, Bo Baslund, and Michael H. Alderman, "Compared With Usual Sodium Intake, Low- and Excessive-Sodium Diets Are Associated With Increased Mortality: A Meta-Analysis," *American Journal of Hypertension* 27, no. 9 (September 2014): 1129–37.

227 M. H. Alderman et al., "Low Urinary Sodium Is Associated With Greater Risk of Myocardial Infarction Among Treated Hypertensive Men," *Hypertension* 25, no. 6 (1995): 1144–52.

228 James J. DiNicolantonio and Sean C. Lucan, "The Wrong White Crystals: Not Salt but Sugar as Aetiological in Hypertension and Cardiometabolic Disease," *Open Heart* 1 (2014): e000167.

B Vitamins

B vitamins—B_1, B_2, B_3, B_5, B_6, B_7, B_9, and B_{12}—play vital roles in metabolism, energy production, and brain health. Because they are water-soluble, B vitamins cannot be stored in the body and must be replenished daily. While synthetic B vitamins are common in supplements and fortified foods, they are often derived from coal tar derivatives and may lack the synergistic effects found in whole food sources.

The most effective way to obtain B vitamins is through nutrient-dense foods that provide the entire B complex in its natural form. Bee pollen and grass-fed beef liver are two of the richest natural sources. For those unable (or unwilling) to consume fresh liver, desiccated beef liver pills are a convenient alternative.

Critical Trace Minerals

While macrominerals such as sodium, magnesium, and potassium are essential in large amounts, trace minerals are equally critical in smaller amounts. Depleted soils, environmental toxins, and modern lifestyle factors necessitate a focus on the following vital trace minerals:

Iodine. Essential for the production of thyroid hormone, iodine supports the metabolic rate of every cell in the body. The best food-based source is seaweed (e.g., kelp, nori, dulse), but other seafood, dairy products, and eggs can help support healthy iodine levels.

Copper. We've already discussed the importance of getting plenty of bioavailable copper, but it's also one of the minerals that has seen the greatest decline in availability from modern foods. The best sources are organ meats (e.g., liver, kidney), shellfish (e.g., oysters, crab), cocoa, nuts (e.g., cashews, almonds), seeds, and whole grains.

Selenium. Critical for thyroid function, antioxidant protection, and immune system support, selenium is also notoriously depleted in our modern soils. The richest source (by far) is Brazil nuts, followed by seafood (e.g., tuna, salmon, sardines), organ meats (e.g., kidney, liver), eggs, and whole grains.

Zinc. While zinc supplementation has its risks, adequate dietary zinc is essential for immune function, wound healing, and enzymatic processes. Key sources include shellfish (e.g., oysters, crab), red meat, poultry, nuts, seeds (e.g., pumpkin, hemp, sesame), and dairy.

Boron. Although not always recognized as essential, boron is essential for balancing key hormones (such as estrogen, testosterone, and vitamin D), supporting magnesium absorption, and promoting bone health. It also reduces oxidative stress caused by heavy metals and environmental toxins. A wide variety of quality fruits, vegetables, nuts, and legumes should provide enough boron, but supplementing with 1–3 mg daily may offer additional benefits in helping to counteract the many assaults of modern life.

Simple, Nutritious Combos

It's surprisingly easy to combine these pillars in ways that are as tasty and convenient as they are healthy.

For example, pickle juice has become popular with athletes as a natural electrolyte supplement. While most pickles are cheaply mass-produced with a vinegar brine, opt for shots of real pickle juice from naturally fermented pickles, which not only provide a dose of salt, but also deliver gut-boosting pre-, pro-, and post-biotics.

Similarly, try dipping homemade sourdough bread in a blend of extra-virgin olive oil and balsamic vinegar to combine the oil's healthy fats and polyphenols with the vinegar's fermented compounds. Add salty olives, aged (fermented) cheeses, naturally cured meats, and perhaps some homemade sprouted chickpea hummus for a complete charcuterie board.

Consider a stir-fry made with grass-fed beef or fermented tofu, cooked in ghee or coconut oil, and loaded with colorful, fiber-rich vegetables like broccoli, bell peppers, and snap peas. Add a splash of tamari, miso, or soy sauce for a dish that hits almost every pillar in one go.

Finally, it's easy to upgrade dessert with a bowl of plain, whole-milk Greek yogurt topped with organic berries, bee pollen, and cacao nibs. This tasty combination brings together a cultured protein source with healthy fats, fiber, and several critical micronutrients.

Conclusion

As we conclude Part Two, it's easy to become discouraged by the many ways in which our dietary staples and mainstream nutritional recommendations seem to oppose God's design for human flourishing. Our store shelves, potlucks, and pantries are flooded with ultra-processed food-like substances that we largely subsidize with our own tax dollars, and it can be difficult to imagine the alternative to this deeply ingrained way of life.

Nevertheless, there is a growing movement toward the recognition that *real* food is the answer, largely centered on five key pillars that bear witness to the logic of God's design: quality protein, natural fats, fiber, fermented foods, and key micronutrients. Eliminating or significantly reducing the primary drivers of metabolic dysfunction may be the most challenging first step for many, but replacing them with these pillars is becoming easier than ever.

In Part Three, we'll build upon this foundation by refining our Christian approach to nutrition, delving into the biblical perspective on some intriguing and even controversial topics. We'll transcend mere questions of what to eat, embracing a comprehensive framework in which food serves as just the beginning of a deeper, more holistic understanding of nourishment and the Christian life on earth.

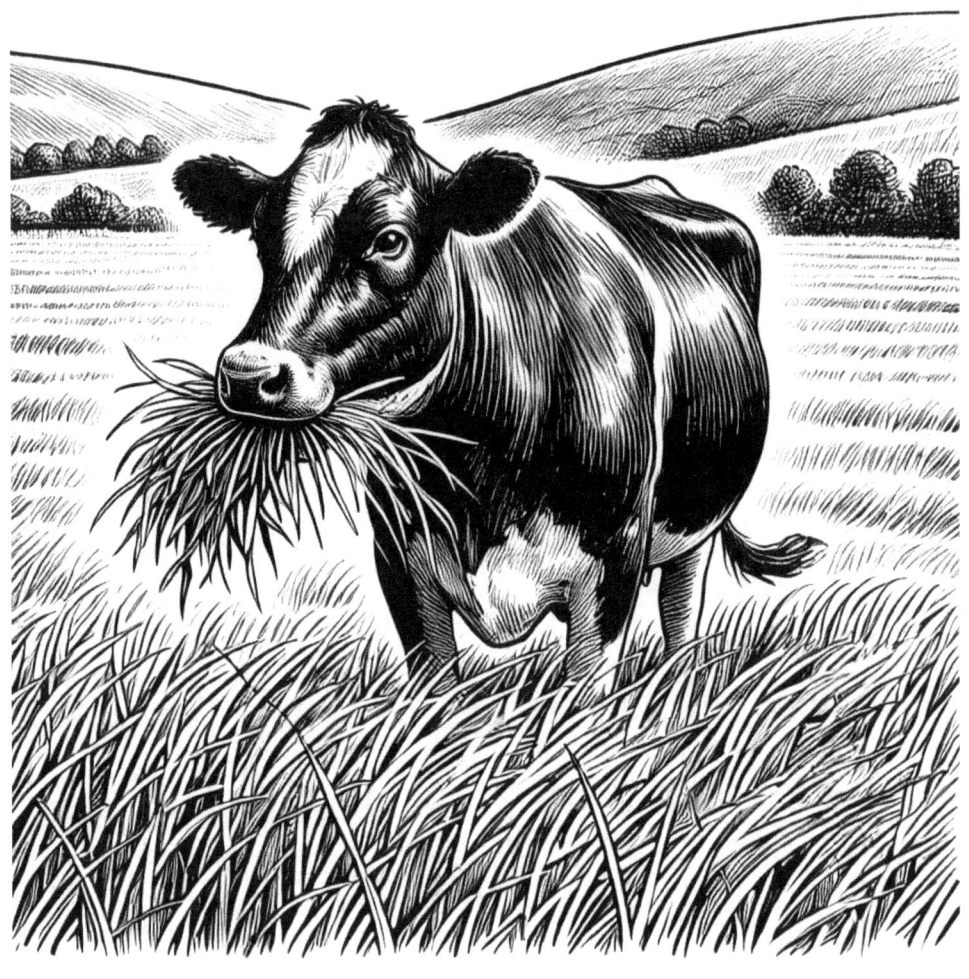

PART III

Refining the Paradigm (Eating with Intention)

"So, whether you eat or drink, or whatever you do, do all to the glory of God."

– 1 Corinthians 10:31

Ⓐll animals eat. Humans, however, are the only creatures who struggle with the question, "How *should* we eat?" Unlike other animals, our appetites are not limited to the actual, the pleasant, or the useful. While we share these basic drives, we are also drawn to higher aspirations: the true, the good, and the beautiful.

As we explored in the section on gratitude and delight in the Eucharistic approach to food (Chapter Three), our relationship with food should involve more than mere utility; it should invite us to recall God's abundant provision and participate in His creative order. In other words, we are the only creatures for whom the animalistic need for food can and should be directed toward higher expressions of being that satisfy our appetite for more than food—but for God Himself.

This perspective provides a bridge as we shift gears from Part Two's focus on the useful—nutrients, metabolic health, and the mechanics of food—to refining a Christian paradigm for nutrition that embraces the higher considerations shaping our dietary choices. Entire books could be written on these considerations. For example, Christian hospitality transforms the table into a place of service and fellowship, welcoming strangers and uniting family and friends. Cultivating civility through table etiquette is also worth exploring as a way of demonstrating and perfecting our best human tendencies.[229] In this section, however, we will focus on several spiritual and ethical issues related to food that are particularly relevant—or potentially controversial—for Christians today.

In Chapter Nine, we will rediscover the cycles of feasting and fasting that were once integral to the Christian way of life, shaping our eating patterns to both celebrate God's self-offering abundance and cultivate temperance and spiritual growth. This discussion will emphasize not only the importance of fasting, but also how to fast *effectively*, aligning the practice with the metabolic principles outlined earlier to achieve holistic benefits for both body and spirit.

---

229 Leon Kass has expanded upon some of these topics in his phenomenal book, *The Hungry Soul.*

Next, we'll turn to the topic of animal consumption, which warrants special attention. Prominent Christian health paradigms, such as the "Genesis Diet," often advocate the avoidance of meat and align with broader societal trends that promote a plant-based diet as morally superior. This anti-meat narrative has significantly influenced Western dietary patterns over the past century, as noted in the Introduction. But is abstinence from meat really a biblically inspired goal? Chapter Ten will argue that the anti-meat bias stems from a simplistic and flawed interpretation of Scripture. In contrast, we'll explore a more nuanced and biblically grounded approach to the consumption of meat and animal products.

Finally, in Chapter Eleven, we'll turn our attention to food systems and the ethical concerns involved in putting food on the table, emphasizing the importance of a distinctly Christian approach to environmental stewardship. Expanding on the ethical aspects of animal consumption, we'll challenge the common belief that livestock are inherently harmful to sustainability. In reality, certain animals are essential to regenerative, eco-friendly food systems that can effectively nourish the global population. These systems also prioritize nutrient density, perfectly complementing the metabolic health principles central to this book.

9

Feasting and Fasting (Rediscovering Biblical Food Rhythms)

"It took only one taste of my wife's first batch
to make me realize that I could not go on as a
dieter. Spaetzle exude substantiality: A man who
takes a small helping is a man without eyes to see
what is in front of him. Accordingly, I passed my
plate back for seconds and then thirds, and made
a vow then and there to walk more, to split logs
every day and, above all, to change my religion
from the devilish cult of dieting to the godly
discipline of fasting. I have never regretted it. To
eat nothing at all is more human than to take a
little of what cries out for the appetite of a giant."

– ROBERT FARRAR CAPON, THE SUPPER OF THE LAMB

A biblical approach to nutrition extends beyond questions of *how* and *what* to eat; it also invites us to reflect on *when* to eat and, equally, *when not* to eat. Given God's rhythmic design as seen in the natural cycles of days, weeks, and seasons, we're reminded in Ecclesiastes 3:1 that there is "a time for every purpose under heaven"

(NKJV). This rhythm should be reflected in our eating habits, which are also meant to follow a cadence.

Ecclesiastes 5:18 celebrates the goodness of enjoying food and drink as part of one's daily labor: "Behold, what I have seen to be good and fitting is to eat and drink and find enjoyment in all the toil with which one toils under the sun the few days of his life that God has given him, for this is his lot." But Scripture also points to the value of fasting. Jesus Himself fasted for 40 days and taught His followers that while feasting was more appropriate in His presence, they would one day fast in anticipation of His return.[230]

While modern Western culture encourages eating around the clock, reconnecting with traditional patterns of fasting—daily, weekly, and seasonal—offers profound benefits for the mind, body, and spirit. Deeply rooted in historic church traditions, these practices promise practical and spiritual nourishment by aligning us more closely with the rhythms intended in creation.

The Loss of Christian Fasting in the West

Fasting was central to early and historic Christian Church practice, as evidenced by the writings of early Church Fathers such as Tertullian, Clement of Alexandria, and Origen. The historical church calendar was heavily influenced by corporate fasting practices, many of which will be explored in this chapter. But while the Eastern Orthodox Church has preserved at least some vestige of these traditions, Western Christians have largely abandoned them.

As Charles Murphy, a Roman Catholic priest and theologian, recalls, Pope John Paul II once remarked during a visit to America in 1980, "What happened to fasting and abstinence in the Church in the United States?"[231] It didn't take long for the pope to realize that the

---

230 Matthew 9:14–15.

231 Charles Murphy, *The Spirituality of Fasting: Rediscovering a Christian Practice* (Notre Dame, IN: Ave Maria Press, 2010) (as cited in Jay W. Richards, *Eat, Fast, Feast: Heal Your Body While Feeding Your Soul—A Christian Guide to Fasting* [San Francisco: HarperOne, 2020]).

Lenten calendar in America was (and remains) essentially a watered-down relic or symbol without much of its historical substance. Today, for Western Catholics, the Code of Canon Law requires only an hour of fasting before Communion, abstinence from meat on Fridays during Lent, and two days of fasting—Ash Wednesday and Good Friday—where even the definition of "fasting" allows for a full meal and two small snacks.[232]

Protestant fasting practices, while less uniform, generally follow the lead of the Swiss reformer Ulrich Zwingli. In 1522, Zwingli defended those arrested for eating dried sausage during Lent—a controversy later dubbed the "Affair of the Sausages." While certainly not opposed to fasting itself, Zwingli correctly noted that fasting is not commanded in Scripture and invoked the doctrine of sola scriptura to defend Christian freedom against the elevation of human laws and traditions to the level of divine law.[233] He summarizes his position in a sermon that has become emblematic of Protestant fasting doctrine ever since: "If you will fast, do so; if you do not wish to eat meat, eat it not; but leave Christians a free choice in the matter." By reclassifying fasting from a matter of law to a matter of personal freedom, many Protestants have abandoned the practice altogether.

Are Roman Catholics, with their diminished Lenten calendar, and Protestants, who largely emphasize Christian liberty at the expense of corporate fasting, missing out on the spiritual and physical benefits of this rich tradition?

Although fasting has largely disappeared from Christian practice, it has recently experienced a resurgence in unexpected places. As modern science confirms its efficacy as a potent form of medicine, fasting has become central to the "biohacking" trend—the practice of manipulating biology to enhance human performance.

---

232 *Code of Canon Law (as cited in Richards, Eat, Fast, Feast).*

233 Russell P. Johnson, "The Affair of the Sausages and Religious Freedom," *The University of Chicago Divinity School*, accessed September 4, 2024, https://divinity.uchicago.edu/sightings/articles/affair-sausages-and-religious-freedom.

Nowhere is this more evident than in Silicon Valley, where leaders of the tech world have traded the indulgent lifestyles of past elites for a disciplined, monk-like ethic aimed at maximizing mental and physical performance. Twitter founder Jack Dorsey, for instance, adheres to a one-meal-a-day regimen and extends his fasting on weekends. In these circles, cutting-edge biohacking strategies that leverage the body's innate survival instincts to optimize cognitive abilities, energy levels, and longevity are par for the course.

However, this biohacking movement diverges significantly from Christian asceticism. Whereas traditional Christian ascetics viewed the body as a sacred gift to be offered back to God, many biohackers view it as raw material to be sculpted according to their desires. Many practitioners of this lifestyle have shifted the motivation for fasting from its original purpose of aligning one's will with the divine will to maximizing worldly gain and relentlessly prolonging life. In this quest to seize control over mortality, some biohackers lay claim of a temporary reward but paradoxically sacrifice the hope of eternity.

Yet secular fasters may have rediscovered something important. Human survival depended on our ancestors' ability to endure periods of scarcity, a concept foreign to today's culture of perpetual abundance. They didn't have granola bars and fruit juice to maintain their blood sugar, and they certainly didn't subscribe to the modern "six small meals a day" mantra. They fasted either because they had to, or because their culture valued it, or both. When food became available or socially acceptable again, they feasted, not thinking about how many calories they were consuming or whether their "macros" were out of whack. In other words, our ancestors used their metabolisms as God designed them, seamlessly switching between burning glucose and fat for energy.

Could biohackers, with their routines of intermittent fasting, time-restricted eating, and other biologically sound protocols, offer valuable insights that Christians could integrate into a more holistic approach to fasting?

In a world no longer dominated by food scarcity or fasting traditions, reviving this ancient practice could provide profound spiritual and physical benefits by reconnecting us to the rhythms embedded in God's design for human flourishing.

The Benefits of Fasting

Christian fasting underscores the holistic nature of humanity—a unity of body, mind, and spirit. The practice recognizes the creaturely neediness of the body and channels it in service of the soul. At the same time, the spiritual rewards of fasting often manifest in physical benefits, contributing to increased vitality and possibly even longevity.

Secular biohackers who focus solely on physical optimization may overlook crucial aspects of proper fasting. Conversely, some Christians mistakenly believe that a fast that leaves the body feeling revitalized and more energetic lacks the sacrificial essence necessary to qualify in the first place. Throughout church history, heretical movements have perpetuated the notion of pitting the body against the soul, but true Christian fasting rejects this false dichotomy.

As Alexander Schmemann aptly states, "Christian asceticism is a fight, not *against* but *for* the body."[234] Similarly, the Church Father Athanasius emphasized the balanced nature of fasting, preaching, "It is required that not only with the body should we fast, but with the soul."[235]

This perspective was perhaps most profoundly embodied by St. Antony, the ascetic monk whose retreat into the desert in the third century ushered in a golden age of monastic fasting practices. Though Antony's practices didn't exactly match popular comedic depictions of the self-punishing monastic life—in which monks humorously bash each other's heads with wooden planks—he nonetheless subjected his body to a rather harsh regimen, featuring an austere diet and extended periods of fasting. But while these practices may seem reminiscent of

---

234 Alexander Schmemann, *Great Lent: Journey to Pascha* (Crestwood, NY: St. Vladimir's Seminary Press, 1974).

235 Athanasius' First Letter, "Of Fasting, and Trumpets, and Feasts."

Gnostic dualists, his motivation paradoxically reflected a deep reverence for the body and its role in spiritual growth.

For Antony, the desert life was a moral endeavor in which body and soul worked together for mutual reform. As scholar Todd Daly explains, Antony saw fasting as "a moral project in which the body was heavily implicated in the reformation of the soul even as the body also reaped the fruit of the soul's reformation," emphasizing that Antony "sought to bring the soul in submission to God *through* the body, not merely against it."[236] Through this lens, fasting is intended to align both body and soul in submission to God, cultivating self-control and deepening one's appreciation of life as a divine gift.

While Antony emphasized the spiritual significance of fasting, he also acknowledged its physical benefits, believing that it could slow aging and restore a glimpse of the exceptional longevity of the Old Testament patriarchs. Indeed, he succeeded, living to the ripe old age of 105!

Modern science now validates many of the benefits Antony attributed to fasting, including its metabolic advantages, enhancement of mental clarity, and cultivation of self-discipline and virtue.

Fasting as a Metabolic Supercharger

The first of the many benefits of fasting lies in its profound metabolic effects, which go far beyond simply burning fat or lowering blood sugar. Fasting triggers a cascade of hormonal and cellular responses that optimize energy use, repair cellular damage, and improve overall metabolic health. These effects reveal the incredible adaptability of the human body, which is designed to thrive in cycles of feast and famine. Understanding the mechanics of these processes sheds light on why fasting has been a cornerstone of health and vitality for centuries.

As previously discussed, insulin levels rise immediately after eating a meal to help manage the immediate spike in blood sugar, dropping as glucose levels subside. This drop signals the body to tap into its

---

236 Todd Daly, "The New Asceticism: Biohacking the Body for Greater Longevity," *Dignitas* 29, no. 1–2 (2022): 18–22.

stored energy reserves, where glucagon, insulin's counterpart, steps in to stabilize blood sugar between meals. Glucagon instructs the liver to convert stored glycogen into glucose, ensuring a steady supply of blood sugar. At the same time, it triggers the release of free fatty acids from fat stores, providing another important source of energy.

Once these fatty acids reach the liver, some are converted into ketones—molecules that can cross the blood-brain barrier and serve as an alternative or supplemental energy source to sustain cognitive function. In fact, the ketogenic diet, which promotes the continued use of ketones for fuel, was developed in the 1920s because it was found that this brain fuel eliminated seizures in people with epilepsy, a disease of impaired glucose metabolism in the brain. While initially focused on epilepsy, ketogenic research has expanded to explore potential therapeutic benefits for conditions ranging from cancer to cardiovascular disease, further underscoring its relevance to metabolic health.

In addition to serving as brain fuel during fasting, ketones act as powerful signaling molecules that induce positive metabolic changes throughout the body. High ketone levels send the signal that times are lean and trigger a cellular program of stress resistance and detoxification. For example, ketones, just like the SCFA butyrate, promote mitochondrial uncoupling, where mitochondria generate heat instead of ATP. As previously discussed, this protective mechanism, while seemingly wasteful, prevents mitochondria from becoming overworked, reduces ROS production, and decreases oxidative stress. This explains why ketones are often referred to as cellular antioxidants.[237]

In addition to detoxifying and preserving mitochondrial function, fasting also slows cell growth and promotes a crucial process known as autophagy, in which cells undergo deep maintenance and cleansing. Critical for optimizing the body's function during times of scarcity, autophagy allows cells to rejuvenate themselves by recycling damaged organelles, proteins, and membranes to ensure they remain healthy and functional. While stimulating cell growth is important for tissue repair

---

237 Pedro Rojas-Morales et al., "Ketone Bodies, Stress Response, and Redox Homeostasis," *Redox Biology* 29 (2020): 101395.

and regeneration, balancing growth with regular autophagy is critical for maintaining overall health. This cellular "spring cleaning" reduces inflammation, improves insulin sensitivity, and clears damaged cells, ultimately reducing the risk of chronic disease and promoting longevity.

Autophagy kicks in when the cell senses three conditions at the same time:

1. Insulin must be low and glucagon high, which typically occurs shortly after the body processes carbohydrates and protein from a meal.

2. Mechanistic Target of Rapamycin (mTOR)—a cellular growth molecule sensitive to the amino acid leucine—must be suppressed, which typically occurs about 12–24 hours after protein ingestion.

3. AMP-activated kinase (AMPK), which acts like a reverse cellular fuel gauge, must be elevated. When cellular energy is low, AMPK boosts mitochondrial function to meet energy demands.

These triggers demonstrate why fasting is a reliable trigger for autophagy. While ketogenic diets that limit carbohydrates and protein promote low insulin and mTOR levels (flipping two of the three switches), AMPK is only significantly elevated by fasting or exercise. Approximately 12–18 hours into a fast, these three cellular switches begin to align themselves in such a way as to promote autophagy, peaking after approximately 24–48 hours of fasting.

By promoting ketone production and autophagy, fasting acts as a powerful tool for metabolic cleansing and quality control, offering profound improvements in overall metabolic health.

Fasting for Clarity

The next major benefit of fasting is its well-documented ability to enhance mental clarity.

It's very unlikely that anyone has ever reported being in peak mental condition after a heavy Thanksgiving meal. On the contrary, improved concentration, sharper focus, and better overall cognitive performance are often reported during extended periods of fasting. This makes sense—why would God design the body to experience mental fog during times of food scarcity? While the idea may seem foreign in an age of food abundance, our ancestors required heightened mental acuity to secure food during lean times. So, while some fear that fasting dulls the senses, medical studies show the opposite,[238] as do the testimonies of faithful fasters throughout church history.[239]

Biologically speaking, this phenomenon has been largely attributed to the neuroprotective effects of ketones. In addition to their role as an alternative energy source for the brain and a potent cellular antioxidant, ketones promote epigenetic changes that increase levels of brain-derived neurotrophic factor (BDNF). BDNF is essential for brain plasticity, neuronal maintenance, and improved learning and memory. During fasting, elevated levels of BDNF may enhance mental clarity, paving the way for deeper prayer, more focused contemplation of Scripture, and a richer spiritual experience.

But beyond the biological benefits, fasting frees up time normally spent preparing and eating meals, allowing these new neural pathways to be filled with Scripture. Renowned Christian professor Peter Kreeft summarizes this idea by suggesting, "In order to create time to pray, we must destroy time to do something else. We must kill something, refuse

---

238   Harris R. Lieberman et al., "A Double-Blind, Placebo-Controlled Test of 2 d of Calorie Deprivation: Effects on Cognition, Activity, Sleep, and Interstitial Glucose Concentrations," *The American Journal of Clinical Nutrition* 88, no. 3 (2008): 667–76.

239   Some might be skeptical of this claim, given the widespread personal experience of feeling irritable or "hangry" after not eating for even just a few hours. This, unfortunately, is the result of a dysfunctional metabolism. Learning how to fast *effectively* and in a way that allows us to harness the mental benefits of fasting is something we'll discuss later in this chapter.

something, say no to something."[240] By occasionally saying no to food, we create space to say yes to spiritual nourishment—through devotions, prayer, meditation, or Scripture reading, for example—aligning the biological benefits of fasting with a deeper walk with God.

The cognitive benefits of fasting—driven by the brain's use of ketones and the additional time for spiritual growth—can feel immediately rewarding. But it's the cumulative effects that yield long-term benefits. Routine fasting promotes lasting metabolic changes that help prevent disease, especially cognitive disease. In fact, impaired autophagy in the brain is being investigated as a prime contributor to neurodegenerative diseases in old age.[241] This offers strong support for the idea that habitual fasting can significantly improve mental clarity and cognitive function, not only for the duration of the fast, but throughout life.

Fasting for Virtue

Finally, beyond its metabolic and cognitive benefits, fasting serves as a powerful tool for cultivating virtue and bringing one's desires under the control of a properly ordered will. Fasting is one of the best ways to cultivate the cardinal virtue of temperance, which provides a powerful defense against the sin most directly related to consumption: gluttony.

At its core, gluttony embodies a disordered desire for food—excessive indulgence, a lack of moderation, and an unquenchable craving for sensory gratification. Just as Western churches have witnessed a decline in the practice of fasting, there is a widespread perception that gluttony has become a socially acceptable sin. How many modern churches harbor compulsive overeaters who are never given a word of rebuke? Perhaps this is because, while some display this sin more visibly

---

240 Peter Kreeft, *Time*, accessed September 4, 2024, https://www.peterkreeft.com/topics/time.htm.

241 Mark P. Mattson, Valter D. Longo, and Michelle Harvie, "Impact of Intermittent Fasting on Health and Disease Processes," *Ageing Research Reviews* 39 (October 2017): 46–58.

than others, it's a struggle that touches far closer to home for most of us—even the fittest—than we care to admit.

We are all prone to wanting more, seeking a greater portion, or blurring the line between hard-earned enjoyment and indulgent excess. In modern America, our abundant provision and cultural inclination to upsize everything make the temptation of gluttony especially difficult to resist.[242] Yet despite its diminished emphasis, the inherent deadliness of gluttony remains unchanged. Gluttony impairs our ability to appreciate God's gifts—especially food—by enslaving us to disordered desires.

The root of gluttony lies in the natural hunger with which all people are born. As we discussed in the Introduction, this hunger is not a design flaw. Therefore, attempting to suppress or ignore it would do nothing but leave us hopeless and frustrated. Instead, our physical hunger is intended to point to a more holistic hunger—one that seeks what is truly satisfying.

Conventional wisdom teaches that overcoming addictions or disordered desires requires redirecting those desires toward something more fulfilling. For example, those who want to quit smoking often succeed not by denying their cravings altogether, but by replacing the habit with healthier behaviors or by focusing on deeper motivations, such as improving their health for the sake of loved ones. This is where Christian fasting finds its purpose—not merely in curbing our physical hunger or denying its existence, but in using it as a powerful means to redirect our longing from mere food to something far greater: a longing for the return of the Bridegroom.

As Christian author Jason Todd writes, "The desire for 'more' is not inherently bad, but is often misdirected. What we need is a relentless appetite for the divine... A taste of His supreme goodness is enough to lure an appetite long held prisoner to lesser portions."[243]

To illustrate this idea, consider this profound discourse between Jesus and His followers:

---

242 This perception is outlined in Jason Todd, "The Socially Acceptable Sin," *Relevant*, April 16, 2015. https://relevantmagazine.com/faith/socially-acceptable-sin/.

243 Ibid.

Then the disciples of John came to him, saying, "Why do we and the Pharisees fast, but your disciples do not fast?" And Jesus said to them, "Can the wedding guests mourn as long as the bridegroom is with them? The days will come when the bridegroom is taken away from them, and then they will fast. No one puts a piece of unshrunk cloth on an old garment, for the patch tears away from the garment, and a worse tear is made. Neither is new wine put into old wineskins. If it is, the skins burst and the wine is spilled and the skins are destroyed. But new wine is put into fresh wineskins, and so both are preserved." (Matt. 9:14–17)

Jesus emphasized that while fasting was by no means a new practice during His ministry, it would take on a whole new character in light of His coming, death, and resurrection. John Piper further explains this idea, clarifying the metaphor of new wine in old wineskins to emphasize Jesus's broader message that fasting should be directed toward cultivating a proper hunger:

"One of the meanings of Christian fasting is that we are expressing our hunger for the Lord Jesus to come back and to take up his kingship in this world. What sets Christian fasting apart as unique—new wine that can't fit into the old wineskins—is that Christ has already come. The Bridegroom, the King, has already been here. We have seen him and known him. We love him, because we have tasted of his presence. We have already tasted the presence of the kingship of Jesus."[244]

This sets the tone for fasting as an expression of longing and hope, rather than a burdensome ritual.

But Jesus also warned that fasting could easily lose its spiritual significance when done for superficial reasons:

"And when you fast, do not look gloomy like the hypocrites, for they disfigure their faces that their fasting may be seen by

244 John Piper, "Why Do Christians Fast?" *Desiring God*, February 8, 2016.

others. Truly, I say to you, they have received their reward. But when you fast, anoint your head and wash your face, that your fasting may not be seen by others but by your Father who is in secret. And your Father who sees in secret will reward you." (Matt. 6:16–18)

In these verses, Jesus counsels against presenting an unkempt or deliberately degrading appearance while fasting, seeking sympathy or admiration; instead, he urges fasters to maintain a composed demeanor and quietly appreciate the opportunity.

St. Basil the Great adds an exclamation point to this idea, saying,

"No one is passionless when he is receiving a victory crown! No one is gloomy when a victory monument is being erected for him. Don't make being healed gloomy! It's outrageous that you don't rejoice over the health of your soul, but grieve over changing foods."[245]

All of these passages point to the proper purpose of fasting: to cultivate an orderly hunger and thus to nurture the virtue of self-control in all things.

But while fasting for virtue may seem primarily a spiritual practice, Antony's example highlights the profound role of the body in transforming disordered desires. Fasting harmonizes hormonal activity, enhances the body's ability to burn fat for energy, and gives the taste buds a much-needed respite from the relentless stimulation of intense, often artificial flavors.

This recalibration is strikingly evident when one cuts out sugary foods. After fasting or a period of reduced sugar consumption, people often find that their perception of taste shifts, suddenly noticing the natural sweetness in carrots, bell peppers, or other foods that once seemed bland. Such moments of rediscovery highlight how fasting can attune us to the simple, unadulterated sweetness of God's provision—a tangible reminder of His self-offering love.

---

245 St. Basil the Great's First Homily on Fasting

Though most obvious with sweetness, fasting reorients the entire metabolic system, sharpening the body's hunger and satiety cues. Ultimately, it reshapes our relationship with food, grounding it in gratitude and moderation rather than excess or compulsion, and assisting in the cultivation of virtue and a well-ordered hunger in all areas of life.

Implementing Rhythms of Fasting and Feasting

Given the manifold benefits of balancing our feasting with fasting, it's important to consider what this rhythm looks like in practice. In keeping with both our physical design and the traditions of the historic Christian calendar, we can reap the benefits of daily, weekly, and even seasonal food rhythms.

Daily Rhythms

The first rhythm to which we should strive to align our feasting and fasting habits is the body's circadian rhythm. This intricate system, essentially our internal 24-hour clock, helps synchronize metabolic processes with the earth's daily cycle of light, temperature, and nutrient availability.

At the center of this system is the brain's master clock, which relies on visual input from the eyes to synchronize the body's internal clocks with the external light-dark cycle. In turn, peripheral organs, such as the liver, pancreas, and adipose tissue, maintain their own circadian rhythms and communicate with the master clock through a sophisticated network of signaling pathways. This synchronization drives a rhythmic pattern of gene expression that is regulated by epigenetic factors. In fact, a whopping 80 percent of protein-coding genes are expressed cyclically, orchestrating our behavior, physiology, and metabolism in sync with the world around us.[246]

Two key hormones—cortisol and melatonin—help orchestrate these rhythms. Cortisol, often called the "stress hormone," peaks in the morning, triggering the cortisol awakening response (CAR), which promotes alertness and signals the liver to start pumping out glucose in preparation for activity. As the day progresses, cortisol levels decline, paving the way for melatonin production in the evening.

Melatonin not only signals the body to prepare for sleep by regulating the sleep-wake cycle, but also plays a crucial role in metabolic regulation by telling the pancreas to stop producing insulin. This reduction in insulin production helps align the body's metabolic processes with its resting state, ensuring that energy stored earlier in the day is utilized overnight.

In essence, both cortisol and melatonin have the side effect of promoting insulin resistance. As a result, our circadian hormonal shifts create a daily cycle of insulin sensitivity that peaks in the late morning to early afternoon (when levels of both hormones are low), gradually decreases toward the evening, and reaches its lowest point at night.[247]

The circadian rhythm is not a fixed entity, but rather a dynamic one that can be shaped by our lifestyle choices. Aligning sleep, activity, and eating patterns with these rhythms strengthens them, while disrupting them can lead to metabolic dysfunction. In particular, the daily timing of food intake is the largest contributor to setting the circadian rhythms of all peripheral organs, making daily feasting and fasting cycles essential for optimal health.[248]

To optimize this daily rhythm, there's value in ensuring a long, consistent daily fasting period—the time between the last calorie

---

246 Emily N. C. Manoogian et al., "Time-Restricted Eating for the Prevention and Management of Metabolic Diseases," *Endocrine Reviews* 43, no. 2 (September 2021): 405–36.

247 Eleonora Poggiogalle et al., "Circadian Regulation of Glucose, Lipid, and Energy Metabolism in Humans," *Metabolism* 84 (July 2018): 11–27.

248 Manoogian et al., "Time-Restricted Eating for the Prevention and Management of Metabolic Diseases."

consumed in the evening and the first calorie consumed the next day. This may seem counterintuitive, as conventional health advice favors eating many small meals and snacks around the clock to boost metabolism and prevent fat storage. However, science tells a different story: frequent snacking keeps insulin elevated, which, as we know, blocks the ability to burn fat. Extending the fasting period allows insulin to drop, enabling the body to burn glycogen and fatty acids while preserving muscle through increased human growth hormone levels.[249]

Unlike the modern practice of continuous grazing, true feasting and fasting follow the "time-restricted eating" model, which involves limiting caloric intake to a consistent window each day, typically spanning eight to ten hours (no more than twelve hours), and fasting for the remaining time. This method not only begins to unlock some of the benefits associated with more prolonged fasting, such as depleting the body's glycogen stores and promoting a fat-burning state, but also offers other significant benefits, such as improving circadian rhythms, improving insulin sensitivity, reducing oxidative stress and inflammation, and lowering blood pressure.

What's more, all of these benefits are achieved even when total daily energy consumption remains the same![250] A 2019 study demonstrated this effect in eleven overweight people who practiced time-restricted eating for just four days. When their meals were limited to a six-hour window, their fasting glucose, fasting insulin, post-meal glucose spikes, and average glucose levels were significantly lower than when they consumed the same foods spread out over a longer period of time.[251]

Chelsea Blackbird, known as the Christian Nutritionist, sums up so much of the Christian paradigm for nutrition in the mantra, "Eat with the Son and with the sun." We now know the importance

---

249   Jason Fung, "Fasting and Growth Hormone Physiology – Part 3," *The Fasting Method*, September 19, 2023.

250   Manoogian et al., "Time-Restricted Eating for the Prevention and Management of Metabolic Diseases."

251   Edward F. Sutton, Courtney Beyl, J. Allison Early, Paige Cefalu, Eric Ravussin, and Leanne M. Redman, "Early Time-Restricted Feeding Improves Insulin Sensitivity, Blood Pressure, and Oxidative Stress Even without Weight Loss in Men with Prediabetes," *Nutrients* 11, no. 6 (2019): 1234, https://doi.org/10.3390/nu11061234.

of Eucharistic eating, reflected in the first part of her phrase, but we can easily overlook the fundamental importance of eating only during daylight hours whenever possible, a rule of thumb that helps promote a form of time-restricted eating in alignment with our circadian biology.[252]

Is Breakfast Really the Most Important Meal of the Day?

The breakfast debate inspires strong convictions on both sides. To be pedantic, "break-fast" is simply the first meal after an overnight fast, whether eaten at 8 a.m., 10 a.m., or noon; yet in practice most of us picture a morning plate.

Eating a morning meal can be beneficial by helping to stimulate muscle protein synthesis early in the day, helping to achieve a daily protein goal, promoting satiety, and aligning with peak morning insulin sensitivity. Others postpone eating, citing benefits such as mental clarity, reduced cravings, shorter eating windows, and perhaps even a lower overall caloric intake.

There's no universally "right" time to break the overnight fast, but what matters most is getting sunlight exposure and engaging in physical movement, if possible, before the first meal, as these habits help maintain a healthy circadian rhythm. Meal composition matters, too. Most people—especially those who are sedentary or insulin-resistant—do best avoiding refined, concentrated carbohydrates such as cereal, pancakes, and orange juice, which trigger blood-sugar spikes and crashes. A protein- and fat-rich breakfast instead sets a stable, energizing tone. By contrast, highly active individuals or morning exercisers can often tolerate—and even benefit from—some whole-food carbohydrates (e.g., fruit or oats) to replenish glycogen.

Eating within one to four hours of waking suits most lifestyles, though timing is flexible. Until then, start the day with generous fluids and

---

252 Of course, while this idea is generally applicable, it may not always be a very practical guideline for those at extreme latitudes with wild seasonal shifts in sunlight availability.

minerals: water, unsweetened tea, or black coffee. Anything that raises insulin breaks the fast. [253]

Early Bird Special?

Avoiding late-night eating is more than just old-fashioned advice—it's backed by science.

We've already discussed how melatonin, which starts to be produced about three hours before bedtime, inhibits insulin production, making nighttime a bad time to scarf down a carton of ice cream. What's worse, though, is that eating late can also disrupt the glymphatic system, the brain's waste removal mechanism, which operates during deep sleep. Discovered as recently as 2012, this system removes harmful substances such as amyloid beta and tau proteins, both of which are strongly linked to Alzheimer's and other neurodegenerative diseases. Because glymphatic activity peaks in the first half of the night during slow-wave sleep, late-night meals or alcohol can interfere with this vital process. [254]

Consider adopting an early bird dinner schedule to improve sleep quality, shorten the daily eating window, and get a good "brain wash"!

---

253   Some suggest that drinking caffeine on an empty stomach early in the morning can increase cortisol and adrenaline, potentially leading to elevated stress levels or hormonal imbalance over time. For those concerned about this effect, matcha green tea offers a gentler alternative, as its L-theanine content provides a calming, focused effect that counteracts some of the caffeine's stimulating properties. Others opt for Bulletproof coffee (coffee blended with grass-fed butter and MCT oil), a drink popularized by biohacker Dave Asprey. This blend is thought to extend the fast by maintaining low insulin levels, offering sustained energy and mental clarity through ketone production.

254   Oliver Cameron Reddy and Ysbrand D. van der Werf, "The Sleeping Brain: Harnessing the Power of the Glymphatic System through Lifestyle Choices," *Brain Sciences* 10, no. 11 (November 17, 2020): 868.

Weekly Rhythms

Just as the body follows a daily circadian rhythm, Christian tradition observes a weekly rhythm.

The *Didache*, one of the earliest non-canonical writings of the Church Fathers, sheds light on this pattern: "Let not your fasts be with the hypocrites, for they fast on Mondays and Thursdays, but you shall fast on Wednesdays and Fridays."[255] Who were these "hypocrites"? No one knows for sure, although historical evidence suggests that they were probably devout Jews or members of the broader pagan culture. The author encourages Christians to distinguish their practices from these groups, which were likely seen as performative acts of piety. But regardless of the details, the passage clearly depicts a structured fasting routine in the early church, symbolically aligned with significant days of the week.

Wednesday marks the night of Jesus's betrayal, while Friday marks His crucifixion. Both days were observed as times of repentance, devoted to fasting, prayer, and reflection on the Bridegroom's sacrifice. These fasts typically lasted until sundown, after which only one meal was taken. However, this fasting practice was complemented by a weekly feast observed on Sunday—the day of Jesus's triumph over death in His resurrection. Known as the Lord's Day, it was and still remains a time for community gathering and celebration.

Aligning eating habits with the Christian weekly calendar resonates with the popular "5:2 intermittent fasting" protocol. As the name suggests, this plan involves eating normally for five days and restricting intake or adjusting meal timing on two nonconsecutive days. Known to improve insulin sensitivity and aid in weight loss, it can be more sustainable for many compared to continuous calorie-restricted diets. Once again, the early church was doing it before it was cool!

---

255 Didache, 8.1.

Seasonal Rhythms

Finally, there are notable rhythms of feasting and fasting that transcend daily and weekly patterns and align with significant seasons in the Christian calendar.

Lent is the most prominent and well-defined fasting period, serving as preparation for the celebration of Easter. Traditionally beginning on Ash Wednesday, its origins predate the fourth-century Council of Nicaea, the earliest recorded account of its observance. The forty days of Lent echo the forty days Moses fasted on Mount Sinai, the forty years the Israelites wandered in the desert, and, most importantly, the forty days Jesus fasted in the wilderness before His public ministry. While Christians are not expected to fast for forty consecutive days like Moses or Jesus, there is typically an encouragement to give up something of significance, accompanied by specific fasting days.

Another significant period, though not as widely practiced or standardized as Lent, is the period of preparation leading up to Christmas. Beginning after the feast of St. Andrew, which falls on the Sunday closest to November 30th, the Advent season includes prayer and fasting leading up to Christmas Eve.

Although these seasonal observances have different emphases, they share the theme of preparatory fasting culminating in a feast. Advent anticipates the birth of Christ with joyful expectation, while Lent fosters a spirit of repentance and renewed dependence on God in preparation for the commemoration of His Passion. In both, fasting serves to deepen prayer and spiritual reflection, enhancing the celebration of God's redemptive work and His abiding love.

How to Fast

The decision to embrace traditional Christian food rhythms—daily, weekly, and seasonal patterns of feasting and fasting—is a vital first step. But just as important is the strategy: learning how to incorporate these practices *effectively*. For those with less-than-ideal metabolic health, jumping into a fasting routine would result in unnecessary discomfort or a miserable failure (or perhaps both).

In people with flexible metabolisms, body fat functions as a highly accessible energy reserve that is readily used when glycogen stores are depleted. This is the ideal state for effective fasting practices. However, for most people, excess body fat is anything but accessible. Despite carrying more fat than necessary, their bodies remain stuck in sugar-burning mode, unable to tap into fat stores for energy. It's as if their fat cells have a one-way valve that allows storage but blocks release. As we discussed earlier, this is why many people are both overfed and always hungry.

For someone in this state, even a short eight-hour fast can trigger symptoms of hypoglycemia (low blood sugar), such as headaches, fatigue, and irritability—what some colloquially refer to as being "hangry." While fasting should be sacrificial and mildly uncomfortable in some ways, especially at the beginning, fasting that causes excessive suffering is not Christian fasting. If it feels more like an assault on the body than an energizing and cleansing experience, it's probably much closer to the self-flagellation of Gnostic dualists than to the handmaiden of Christian spiritual discipline.

In an effort to revive the practice of fasting in our overfed yet undernourished society, some pastors and Christian wellness advocates have promoted "juice fasting." The idea is to lower the barrier to entry by allowing unlimited juice while forbidding solid food, which provides almost continuous fuel for the body but without the satisfaction of eating.[256] According to at least one proponent of the strategy, when the hunger pangs and feelings of hypoglycemia creep in, just drink more juice! In this way, juice fasting promises to provide the benefits of fasting despite the consumption of sugar throughout the day. A tempting solution, right? But despite good intentions, this misguided beginner's strategy undermines the very purpose of fasting. It simply masks the root cause of metabolic dysfunction and offers no remedy.

---

256 David Mathis, "A Guide to Christian Fasting," *Desiring God*, December 24, 2023.

This is because, as mentioned above, the only way to effectively fast is to unlock the body's fat stores, and the only way to do that is to reduce insulin levels. Continuous juice infusions provide a constant supply of sugar to the bloodstream, keeping insulin elevated and keeping the body in glucose burning mode indefinitely. This strategy is not only ineffective, but counterproductive, a seemingly entry-level tactic that does nothing but exacerbate insulin resistance, increase hunger, and sabotage even the best of fasting intentions. With this kind of foolish approach, it's not hard to see why people aren't interested in fasting.

The more effective strategy for fostering a fasting-friendly metabolism is to reprogram the body to burn fat. While this doesn't happen overnight, many people have experienced remarkable results by combining intermittent fasting with a very low carbohydrate (ketogenic) diet protocol as a temporary metabolic fix.[257] Lent and Advent offer convenient opportunities for such a routine, pairing our good intentions with a culturally accepted framework to help us achieve them.

Christian author and fasting expert Jay Richards advocates for a 40-day regimen that integrates ketogenic principles and progressively structured intervals of intermittent fasting with the traditional fasting and abstinence periods of the Christian calendar.[258] His approach begins by gradually narrowing the daily eating window to extend fasting periods long enough to deplete glycogen reserves and promote fat utilization. This effect can be enhanced by exercising in a fasted state, a practice that can be slowly and progressively incorporated over time. In addition, a very low carbohydrate diet during this time will keep insulin levels low, promote ketosis, and improve cellular health.

This temporary metabolic reset helps participants transition to a state in which feasting and fasting feel natural. More importantly, it lays

---

257 The key word is "temporary." Some may thrive indefinitely on keto diets (more power to them), but some do not. What's inarguable, however, is the efficacy of the approach as a short-term metabolic fix.

258 See a comprehensive roadmap for this approach in Richards, *Eat, Fast, Feast*. Keep in mind, it's important to consider each person's unique starting point, health conditions, and goals, ideally with the help of an experienced health coach or doctor.

the foundation for embracing fasting as a sustainable Christian lifestyle practice long after the restrictive metabolic cleanse is over.

Conclusion

John Piper succinctly captures the essence of Christian eating rhythms: "Food is good. It is a gift of God, and we glorify God with it in two ways, not just one way. We feast on it with gratitude for God's goodness, and we forfeit food out of hunger for God himself."[259]

In modern societies, where food is available at all hours and in endless variety, the once vibrant rhythms of feasting and fasting—so integral to both church and human history—have effectively flatlined. But as fasting gains renewed attention as a mainstream health practice, it's time for the Church to reclaim this ancient discipline and rediscover its holistic benefits.

Fasting supports optimal metabolic health, sharpens mental clarity, and fosters self-control in all things—perfectly complementing the nutritional principles we've already discussed. It, in turn, becomes much more accessible when built on a solid foundation of Eucharistic feasting, avoiding ultra-processed, chemical-laden food-like substances, and prioritizing the Pillars of the Plate.

As we conclude this chapter with a powerful, potentially transformative tool, we turn our attention to the topic of meat—a topic of ongoing debate both in the world and within the Church.

---

259 John Piper, "Why Do Christians Fast?"

10

Rise, Kill, and Eat (A Biblical Case for Meat)

"In the state of society we now have reached, it is difficult to conceive of a people subsisting merely on bread and vegetables. Such a nation if it existed would certainly be subjected by carnivorous enemies, as the Hindus were, to all who ever chose to attack them. If not it would be converted by the cooks of its neighbors as the Boeotians were, after the battle of Leuctra."

– ANTHELME BRILLAT-SAVARIN,
THE PHYSIOLOGY OF TASTE

Throughout history, Christians have wrestled with the idea of consuming animals, often reflecting broader cultural attitudes while also offering distinct theological perspectives. To understand the role of meat in a Christian dietary paradigm, we must consider how the Church has navigated these influences—sometimes conforming to societal norms, sometimes challenging them, and occasionally shaping them. This historical context is essential as we explore the extent to which eating meat aligns with God's design for human flourishing.

The current push against animal consumption—spanning environmental, ethical, and health concerns—is not a novel development. In fact, skepticism about meat has long been a feature of intellectual and cultural discourse. In the early days of Christianity, many Roman elites, influenced by Pythagorean philosophy, avoided meat. Pythagoras, the famous mathematician and philosopher who lived 500 years before Christ, advocated vegetarianism in part because of his belief in the transmigration of souls. After all, few would enjoy eating a steak if they feared it might be the reincarnation of their great-grandfather! Until recently, vegetarianism was even referred to as the "Pythagorean diet," a testament to his enduring influence.

Adding to these dietary influences, early Christians also grappled with the legacy of Jewish dietary laws, which permitted the consumption of meat but excluded certain species, such as pork and shellfish. For many of Christ's earliest followers, embracing a new, unrestricted approach to food was both uncomfortable and profoundly countercultural.

In this cultural and philosophical milieu, dietary concerns became a significant issue for the early church as it sought to distinguish Christian theology from competing ideologies. By promoting a broadly inclusive approach to eating, the Church rejected pagan dietary restrictions and highlighted the fulfillment of the Mosaic Law in Christ. This emphasis on unity and salvation apart from rigid food laws led to the Church's early rejection of meat prohibitions, underscoring the freedom inherent in the Christian faith.

Church fathers such as Irenaeus of Lyon argued that abstaining from meat showed ingratitude toward God's creation, likening it to abstaining from marriage.[260] This view was shared by other early Christian writers, such as Hippolytus of Rome, who explained that vegetarians abstained from animal flesh "out of pride."[261]

By the thirteenth century, the largely Christian Roman Empire, with few exceptions, was quite supportive of meat consumption.

---

260 Carl Frayne, "On Imitating the Regimen of Immortality or Facing the Diet of Mortal Reality: A Brief History of Abstinence From Flesh-Eating in Christianity," *Journal of Animal Ethics* 6, no. 2 (October 2016): 188–212.

261 Ibid.

Thomas Aquinas, reflecting the medieval mindset, wrote in his *Summa Theologiae*:

> "All animals are for man. Whereof, it is not unlawful if men use ... animals for the good of man ... This cannot be done unless [animals] are deprived of life ... this is in keeping with the commandment of God Himself."[262]

But while historical Christian writings overwhelmingly support meat consumption, vegetarianism has also been endorsed in specific contexts. Clement of Alexandria claimed that the apostle Matthew "partook of seeds, nuts, and vegetables, without flesh,"[263] while also suggesting that meals shared among Christians "should not include the smell of roasting meat."[264] Similarly, church fathers such as Jerome and Basil the Great idealized a vegetarian diet, seeing it as a reflection of humanity's original and heavenly state, which they believed Christians on earth should strive to emulate.[265]

Interestingly, at times, the dietary practices of the most devout and the most heretical Christians were almost indistinguishable, each practicing abstinence from meat. For example, the Cathars, a heretical Christian sect in the Middle Ages, strictly avoided meat. Of course, their strict vegetarianism, like that of other prominent Gnostic dualist sects, did not arise from concern for animal welfare but from a disdain for the material world. In their view, flesh was emblematic of the proliferation of matter and was therefore completely forbidden.

Catholic monasteries also adopted meatless diets, often subsisting on only bread, vegetables, and salt. But while this ascetic diet may have resembled that of their heretical Gnostic counterparts, the motivations behind it were fundamentally different. Monks and nuns didn't despise the material world; rather, they viewed meat as one of God's good gifts and believed that to reject it altogether was a sign of pride. Influenced

---

262 Thomas Aquinas, *Summa Theologiae*, II-I, q. 102, art. 6 (as cited in Frayne, "On Imitating the Regimen of Immortality.").

263 2.1, 16 (as cited in Frayne, "On Imitating the Regimen of Immortality.")

264 Leyerle, 1995, pg. 153 (as cited in Frayne, "On Imitating the Regimen of Immortality.")

265 Frayne, "On Imitating the Regimen of Immortality."

by early Christian ascetic practices, monasteries sought to balance the goodness of an omnivorous diet with the cultivation of self-mastery and a properly ordered will.

To maintain this balance, the Church explicitly sought to ensure that all Christians had a taste for meat, even if they abstained from eating it. Abstinence, the Church argued, could not serve its penitential purpose if there was no desire for meat in the first place. Reflecting this principle, the Second Council of Toledo in 447 declared that anyone who abstained from meat "not in a spirit of bodily mortification but out of disgust" should be excommunicated, as such attitudes aligned with the heretical tendency to despise the flesh rather than honor God's creation.

It's safe to say, then, that historic Christianity has overwhelmingly supported meat consumption as a general theme. Vegetarianism, however, has also been widely accepted and even endorsed as a form of discipline, condemned only when associated with heretical motivations.

But while this pattern has remained largely unchanged for denominations adhering to orthodox Christian beliefs, some smaller offshoots of larger denominations have promoted vegetarianism in recent centuries. For example, the Bible Christian Church and the Liberal Catholic Church have both promoted vegetarianism. Similarly, as noted in the Introduction, Ellen White, the prophetess of the SDA Church, claimed to have received divine visions instructing her to abstain from meat. Her influence on Western dietary attitudes, particularly in shaping vegetarian staple foods and dietary guidelines, is hard to overstate and remains quite powerful.

Interestingly, many modern revivals of Christian vegetarianism have highlighted early arguments largely overlooked in the Middle Ages, suggesting that vegetarianism was God's original design and promoting its supposed health benefits. Because these claims are both popular and influential, this chapter will address them with the goal of developing a theology of meat that is more consistent with Scripture and the broader Christian tradition.

As we do so, however, we should remember that dietary debates were anticipated in Scripture. The apostle Paul specifically foresaw and warned against allowing dietary preferences to cause divisions within the church and needlessly lead people away from Christ. Sure enough, most of the dietary heresies we witness today and throughout church history have both furthered church divisions and revolved around animal consumption in some way, making the resolution of this debate as relevant as ever.

Arguments Against Animal Consumption

"The Original Diet Was Vegan, and so is the Heavenly Diet"

Those who make a theological case against eating meat tend to cite the creation account in Genesis. The reasoning is straightforward: if God's original creative intent was "good," then any deviation from it must be, well, not good.

Genesis 1 says, "And God said, 'Behold, I have given you every plant yielding seed that is on the face of all the earth, and every tree with seed in its fruit. You shall have them for food'" (Gen. 1:29). Doesn't this imply that the originally intended diet was a vegan one? This idea is reinforced by God's instruction to Adam in Genesis 2 that he may freely eat of every tree in the garden except the tree of the knowledge of good and evil.[266] After the Fall, this idyllic Edenic diet shifts, but the theme persists when God curses the ground and declares that Adam will eat of the "plants of the field" (Gen. 3:18–19). Therefore, on three occasions in just the first three chapters of the Bible, God is said to have promoted what we would call a vegan diet.

"Not till after the Flood, when every green thing on the earth had been destroyed," says Ellen White, "did man receive permission to eat flesh."

It's important to note, however, that while these chapters never explicitly grant permission to eat meat, they don't forbid it either. This omission leaves room for speculation. For example, Adam's son Abel

---

266 Gen 2:16–17

is described as a "keeper of sheep" (Gen 4:2). While Abel's flock was probably used for wool, hides, and sacrificial worship, it's not a stretch to speculate that it was also a source of meat and milk. This is consistent with the understanding of sacrifice as a gift of sustenance, where offering a portion of one's food back to the Creator reflects both gratitude and dependence on God. In this context, Abel's use of livestock for basic sustenance seems at least plausible.

The Creation account also raises important questions about the diets of animals. In Genesis, we are told that "every green plant" was given as food for "every beast of the earth." But, as we know, some animals are clearly designed to be carnivorous. Every biological feature of a predator—from its camouflage and behavioral instincts to its jaw structure and digestive system—indicates that it is equipped to hunt and consume other animals. This creates a conundrum for the idea of a purely plant-based original creation, as it is hard to imagine lions subsisting on grass or sharks munching on seaweed.

In the same way, human physiology casts further doubt on the idea of an exclusively plant-based ancestral diet. Unlike herbivorous primates, humans are distinctly omnivorous. Our uniquely generalized teeth, relatively short intestines, and highly acidic stomachs are specifically optimized to digest and extract nutrients from both plants and meat. In contrast, herbivorous primates have flat molars, long digestive tracts, and large, complex colons—features specifically designed to accommodate grinding and fermenting fibrous plant matter such as leaves and stems.

So while it's reasonable to imagine the pre-Flood human diet as purely plant-based, there's room for doubt. This uncertainty, however, should not be viewed as a flaw in the biblical narrative. These passages focus on humanity's unique relationship with God and our stewardship of creation, rather than prescribing a universal diet. While they hold important normative value in some aspects of life, interpreting them as a definitive argument for vegetarianism risks oversimplifying their theological and anthropological depth. In short, Christians should approach arguments for plant-based diets rooted in the Creation account with caution, recognizing that the text's primary purpose lies far beyond dietary prescriptions for our fallen condition.

In addition to Genesis, eschatological imagery of the "new creation" is often cited as evidence against God's intention for meat in the human diet. Indeed, some prophetic visions, such as Isaiah's portrayal of peace among natural enemies, seem to support the idea of a meatless existence in heaven:

> "The wolf shall dwell with the lamb, and the leopard shall lie down with the young goat, and the calf and the lion and the fattened calf together; and a little child shall lead them. The cow and the bear shall graze; their young shall lie down together; and the lion shall eat straw like the ox. The nursing child shall play over the hole of the cobra, and the weaned child shall put his hand on the adder's den. They shall not hurt or destroy in all my holy mountain; for the earth shall be full of the knowledge of the LORD as the waters cover the sea." (Isa. 11:6–9)

It is challenging to reconcile the butchering of a cow with such a vision of peaceful harmony among animals.

Similarly, the apostle John's vision in Revelation presents a heavenly state with "no more death" (Rev. 21:4). If death is abolished in the new creation, wouldn't that corroborate Isaiah's prophecy and imply an end to meat consumption?

Influenced by such prophetic imagery, early church figures like Jerome and Basil the Great advocated for vegetarianism as a foretaste of the harmonious, meatless state of the heavenly kingdom.

Yet not all prophetic imagery aligns with a meatless vision of heaven. For example, when Isaiah isn't describing the idyllic harmony between humans and natural predators, he also describes heaven as a banquet of "rich food full of marrow" (Isa. 25:6). Taken literally and according to our present experience, wouldn't this require the death of an animal?

Such passages raise an important question: were these descriptions intended to convey a literal heavenly diet, or were they written to convey incomprehensible spiritual insights using familiar language and concepts?

This question is unlikely to be resolved in our temporal lives. Nevertheless, Scripture provides a glimpse of the resurrected life through the glorified body of Jesus. After His resurrection, Jesus ate fish—a clear indication that eating animal flesh was not incompatible with His perfected form. His ability to eat while also walking through walls underscores the mystery of the redeemed body and cautions against deriving normative dietary rules from incomplete revelations.

Is Fish Meat?

The controversial distinction between fish and meat has its origins not in the Bible or biology, but in Roman Catholic tradition. The distinction arose largely from fasting regulations, which granted a special exemption to fish as a humbler, more accessible food for the coastal peoples of medieval Europe.

Not surprisingly, this allowance became a point of contention for Christians in landlocked regions around the time of the Reformation. Martin Luther famously criticized the Church's arbitrary and seemingly self-serving Lenten rules, which permitted Roman staples like fish and olive oil but banned butter and beef, both ubiquitous staples in Northern Europe. Wealthier Christians often circumvented these prohibitions by buying indulgences or paying spiritual taxes to Rome, further alienating the poor saps in Luther's parish. For Luther and other reformers, this issue was emblematic of deeper doctrinal corruption, making controversies over fish, olive oil, and butter significant in the broader schism of the sixteenth century.[267]

But for our purposes, it's important to note that there is no theological distinction between fish and other animal flesh, so we should consider them as a part of the same category.

---

267   Roos, Dave, "How Butter Fueled the Protestant Reformation," HowStuffWorks.com, August 28, 2017, https://history.howstuffworks.com/historical-events/butter-fueled-protestant-reformation.htm.

In summary, both the Creation account and much of the prophetic imagery of the new creation are intended to provide truths about humanity's origin, nature, and role in God's redemptive plan. But we must be careful not to interpret every biblical description as a prescription for our present, fallen lives, which exist somewhere in between these states. Moreover, viewing God's provision of meat as a concession for sin, much like Deuteronomy 24's allowance for divorce, diminishes the wisdom of His unfolding covenant. Instead of being a tolerable moral downgrade, the introduction of meat marks a positive covenantal development, deeply intertwined with the concept of sacrifice (see Chapter Two). This provision points to Christ, the Lamb of God, whose flesh is "true food." Eating His body is far from a vegan idea, but rather a sacrificial and incarnational reality: in Christ, flesh becomes the very means of communion and redemption. Scripture moves not from purity to compromise but from garden to glory, where sacrifice is fulfilled, not abolished.

"Veggie Burgers are Less Violent"

Another familiar argument against eating meat comes from those who can't stomach the idea of killing animals. However, the intuitive belief that plant-based diets are inherently less violent than those that include meat isn't entirely accurate. Even if it were, that wouldn't necessarily strengthen the theological case for favoring vegetables over meat.

It's undeniable that a juicy ribeye is a direct product of a slaughtered cow, while a cauliflower steak is not directly linked to the death of any animal. In this sense, the sacrifice of animals is a fundamental part of the meat production process.

However, this simple logic obscures key details that highlight how meat production can paradoxically promote more life. Livestock play a vital role in thriving ecosystems during their lifetimes, supporting an abundance of plant, microbial, and animal life. Well-managed pastures, for example, provide habitat for a wide variety of insect and animal species, with livestock playing a symbiotic role. Their manure enriches the soil, promoting biodiversity and even revitalizing degraded land. Thus, while meat production involves animal death, it can also serve as a net contributor to life and ecological health.

Contrast this with modern industrial farming, which not only devastates natural habitats but also perpetuates a cycle of environmental destruction. These operations clear vast tracts of land, often teeming with life, and till it with heavy machinery before drenching it in pesticides and rodenticides. The result is a sterile landscape, where countless creatures are wiped out to produce monocultures of corn, wheat, or soy.

In more sustainable farming systems, the ideal of a bloodless food production model remains elusive. Even the most well-intentioned small-scale organic farms, free of chemical poisons and intense tilling operations, often resort to trapping and killing small mammals and other critters as collateral damage in the pursuit of protecting their crops. Steven Davis, a professor of animal science at Oregon State University, points out that not only are plant-based diets not bloodless, but "several alternative food production models exist that may kill fewer animals than the vegan model."[268] In other words, the notion of a food system entirely free of death is a naïve fantasy held by those disconnected from the realities of agriculture.

Indeed, quantifying both the loss of life and the lost potential for life in food systems is no easy task. But weighing the moral implications can be even more difficult. How do we compare the deaths of thousands of pollinators, insects, and rodents in monoculture farming with the loss of a single cow or chicken?[269] While we tend to have a special affinity for large animals, with which we identify much more closely than, say, an insect, is there any moral basis to suggest that the loss of a hive, or even

---

268 S. L. Davis, "The Least Harm Principle May Require That Humans Consume a Diet Containing Large Herbivores, Not a Vegan Diet," *Journal of Agricultural and Environmental Ethics* 16, no. 4 (2003): 387–94.

269 The logical counterpoint to this line of reasoning is that monocrop production is currently used to feed most industrial livestock, creating a false dichotomy between meat production and monocrop production. This point will be addressed in more depth in the next chapter, as we discuss both current and ideal sources of livestock feed.

a single bee, is any more acceptable? And for that matter, what justifies the death of an onion?

Moreover, the manner of death raises further ethical questions. Is the violent death of an animal in the wild—gruesomely torn apart by predators or slowly succumbing to disease—any less troubling than a quick, humane slaughter by humans? While it may not always be the norm, humans possess a unique capacity to be the most compassionate and deliberate killers on the planet.

Many people turn to secular ethical frameworks when grappling with these issues. For example, famed ethicist Peter Singer's theory of animal rights is based on the purely utilitarian idea of maximizing happiness and minimizing suffering. In this view, an organism's moral status is determined solely by its capacity to experience pleasure and pain, with animals possessing more developed nervous systems having greater moral status than their seemingly less sophisticated counterparts, like smaller critters, microbes, and insects.

But while this logic seems reasonable at first, it's the same rationale Singer uses to defend late-term abortion and infanticide, arguing that fetuses and even some newborns lack self-awareness and future-oriented preferences and therefore have no moral standing. Such reasoning exposes the dangers of unbiblical moral calculations, which often veer into troubling territory. Left to our own devices, our ethical reasoning can echo the hypocrisy of George Orwell's *Animal Farm*, where "All animals are equal, but some animals are more equal than others."[270]

Ultimately, comparing food systems by their impact on animal life is flawed unless approached from a biblical perspective. When God gives people permission to eat meat, it comes with the idea that all life is inherently valuable. Man, the most precious creature, created in the image of God and entrusted with the responsibility of reflecting God's benevolent dominion over the earth, is thus called to minimize unnecessary death and suffering.

---

270 George Orwell, *Animal Farm* (New York: Harcourt, Brace, 1946).

This doesn't mean, however, that violence is completely absent from the order of creation. Indeed, to reject all violence would be to reject the underlying logic of God's good design. As Norman Wirzba explains, to reject this sacrificial pattern of creation is to reject God's terms for creation, where even death bears witness to self-offering love:

"To reject God's gift of another's life and death in the name of a world free of death or suffering would require the erasure of all life, not simply physiological life but also the life of self-offering love."[271]

To bolster this line of reasoning, it's fascinating to note the paradox that many medieval saints exhibited profound compassion for animals, yet there is no evidence that they were vegetarians. St. Francis of Assisi, for example, was known by his earliest biographers to show "great tenderness towards lower and irrational creatures," often referring to them as "brother or sister," no matter how small they were.[272] But that didn't stop some of these special friends from occasionally adorning his plate, leading scholar Carl Frayne to suggest, "in the medieval period, animals were more likely to be butchered by a compassionate Catholic than a disdainful heretic."[273]

In conclusion, the pacifist argument for biblical veganism fails on both practical and theological grounds. Practically speaking, death is an unavoidable aspect of all food production, and agricultural systems that incorporate animal products can paradoxically result in fewer overall deaths and promote greater biodiversity than systems that exclude animal slaughter. We'll delve deeper into these concepts in the next chapter. But more importantly, the attempt to avoid animal death at all costs is fundamentally misguided, leading us away from biblical truths about the nature of sacrifice and redemption within God's design for life.

---

271 Norman Wirzba, *Food and Faith.*
272 Frayne, "On Imitating the Regimen of Immortality."
273 Ibid.

"Plant-Based Diets are Healthier"

Finally, let's address a common and increasingly accepted Christian argument for minimizing or eliminating animal products: the claim that plant-based diets promote better health than those including animal foods. With a theology of health that emphasizes strength for life as a Christian value, this argument, if true, would indeed challenge the role of meat and other animal products in God's design for human flourishing.

But this claim is deeply flawed and needs to be reframed. The healthfulness of a diet doesn't necessarily depend on the extent to which plants or animal products predominate. After all, from strict vegans and vegetarians to carnivores, there are countless examples of healthy people on all parts of the dietary spectrum. Rather, the healthiness of a diet depends on two things: the degree to which it avoids metabolic toxins and the degree to which it prioritizes the Pillars of the Plate.

It's undeniable that an organic salad is a better choice than a couple of hot dogs cured with nitrates, slathered in sugary ketchup, and held in ultra-processed buns. Much of the meat sold in grocery stores and served in restaurants is mass-produced and of questionable quality, raised in industrial systems that prioritize quantity over nutritional value. Ultra-processed lunch meats and sausages, for example, often contain carcinogenic preservatives and fillers.[274] Even minimally processed meats often come from animals raised on pesticide-laden grains and injected with antibiotics and hormones that can be passed on to consumers second-hand. Most industrially produced dairy products are no better, especially after many nutrients are zapped in the pasteurization process, pulverized through homogenization, or combined with harmful additives. It's important to acknowledge that not all animal products are created equal, and in comparing the best vegetarian diets to the worst omnivorous ones, there's merit in the former.

---

274 This isn't true of *all* lunch meats and sausages, however. Many uncured and minimally processed meat products from consciously raised animals can be a great part of a healthy diet.

However, plant-based diets are not without their potential pitfalls. Ultra-processed oils, refined grains and sugars, dyes, pesticide residues, and iron shavings are increasingly common in plant-based foods, and people who adopt such diets often increase their intake of these metabolic toxins.[275] Consumption of animal products has steadily declined over the past 75 years, but the substitutes have been no better. While the fat, sodium, and cholesterol often found in animal products have been relentlessly demonized, ultra-processed plant substitutes have largely filled the void, and rates of chronic disease have skyrocketed.

Brands associated with the SDA Church are emblematic of these changes. John Harvey Kellogg, as introduced earlier, believed that eliminating the consumption of meat and rich foods could help patients control sexual urges. We now know that saturated fat and cholesterol act as essential precursors to sex hormones like testosterone, so replacing the traditional breakfast of eggs and bacon with his Corn Flakes may indeed have helped his cause. Today, however, breakfast cereals dominate store shelves, while fertility clinics struggle to keep up with demand.

The SDA Church was also largely responsible for introducing the paradoxical holy grail of vegan foods—fake meat—to the market. For decades, Loma Linda Foods marketed Nuteena, an early "meatless meat" created by Kellogg that paved the way for modern products such as "Impossible Meat." This current generation of fake meats is much more "meaty" in texture and flavor, often closely resembling the products they seek to imitate. But this requires the inclusion of ultra-processed oils, binders, preservatives, plant protein extracts, and a host of other unpronounceables. Ironically, these products are not only the culmination, but the perfect encapsulation of the modern vegetarian dilemma. By submitting to the dogma that plant-based diets are superior, many people have been duped into buying expensive, ultra-processed foods that are no better than the traditional diets they fled from.

---

275 Beerman, Kathy,. "Do Plant-Based Ultra-Processed Foods Improve the Nutritional Quality of Vegetarian Diets?" *American Society for Nutrition*, January 15, 2021.

The Daniel Diet

The story of Daniel in the Old Testament is often cited by Christians who advocate a vegetarian or vegan lifestyle. In Daniel 1:8–16, he and his friends choose to reject the rich foods of the king's table—presumably the result of idolatrous sacrifices—in obedience to God. To convince his steward that their condition would be no worse, Daniel proposed an experiment, suggesting that after 10 days of eating nothing but vegetables, he and his friends would look healthier than those who ate the king's food. Sure enough, after 10 days on the vegetable-only diet, they were "better in appearance and fatter in flesh than all the youths who ate the king's food."

At first glance, this story might appear to endorse a vegetarian diet. However, it is far less a commentary on specific dietary choices than a profound testament to God's sovereign power and grace toward those who trust in Him. The passage highlights that Daniel and his friends thrived not because of the inherent superiority of a vegetable-only diet, but because of their faithfulness and God's provision. If anything, the passage implies that it takes divine intervention to achieve health and vitality on a strictly plant-based diet!

Acknowledging that a healthy diet can take many forms and that both plant and animal foods have potential pitfalls, it's essential to recognize the undeniable nutritional advantages of including animal products. Biological anthropologists widely agree that humans are distinctly omnivorous, with a natural preference for meat and other animal products when available. This is supported not only by our anatomical design, as previously discussed, but also by the challenges and nutritional limitations inherent in sustaining an exclusively plant-based diet.

For example, the feasibility of a well-rounded diet without animal products often hinges on modern, first-world conveniences. Unlike animal products, which have historically been available year-round in a variety of climates and economic conditions, a varied vegan diet often relies on global trade and refrigerated transportation. Without these, foods like strawberry-banana protein smoothies or mixed green salads would be seasonal luxuries, available only briefly in cooler climates. While those with access to such resources are free to enjoy them, it raises a broader point: if God intends His people to inhabit all corners of the earth, it seems unlikely that His design for human flourishing would rely on a nutrition model so fragile in its infrastructure and so unique to the modern era. After surveying the dietary habits and health outcomes of dozens of remote and traditional cultures, Weston A. Price observed that "none of them were vegetarian. In every instance they obtained animal proteins and animal fats from some source, and these were highly prized."[276] His findings reinforce the practicality and universality of omnivorous diets, which align more closely with the natural availability of food in a fallen world.

Another key point is that omnivorous diets are especially well-suited to achieving the nutrient density emphasized by the Pillars of the Plate. In contrast, plant-based diets often lack several essential nutrients and require meticulous planning and supplementation to ensure long-term viability. Of course, the severity of this issue varies considerably between vegetarians and vegans. Vegetarians who consume animal-derived products like milk, kefir, aged cheeses, and eggs can generally meet their nutritional needs without extensive supplementation. For strict vegans, however, achieving adequate nutrient intake becomes quite impractical—if not nearly impossible—particularly for nutrients such as vitamin B_{12}, protein, retinol, essential minerals, and omega-3 fatty acids.[277]

Vitamin B_{12}. Vitamin B_{12} deficiency is arguably the most serious and well-documented deficiency of plant-based diets. While B_{12} is abundant in animal products (especially meat and organs), it's almost completely absent from plant-based diets, where the microorganisms that produce it are largely eliminated by modern sanitation processes.

---

276 Weston A. Price, Nutrition and Physical Degeneration (La Mesa, CA: Price-Pottenger Nutrition Foundation, 2008), 295.

277 Joshua Gibbs, and Francesco P. Cappuccio, 2024, "Common Nutritional Shortcomings in Vegetarians and Vegans," *Dietetics* 3, no. 2: 114–128.

Research shows that vegans tend to have fewer traditional risk factors for heart disease, such as high blood pressure and body weight, than omnivores. However, this hasn't consistently translated into lower rates of cardiovascular disease or mortality, with low B_{12} levels emerging as a key independent risk factor for heart disease. Even vegetarians who consume eggs and dairy products may have difficulty avoiding this deficiency.[278]

Protein. Protein deficiency is another notorious challenge associated with plant-based diets. Vegans reflexively counter this common criticism by pointing out that all essential amino acids can be found in plants, with the most abundant sources being leafy greens, nuts, legumes, and grains. However, most plant proteins are incomplete, lacking at least one of the nine essential amino acids. Even the few complete plant protein sources, such as quinoa, tofu, and buckwheat, fall short of the amino acid profiles needed for efficient muscle protein synthesis. Remember, it's not just about consuming enough protein; what truly matters is the delivery of the necessary amino acids to the cells in the right ratios. This forces vegans to carefully combine different plant proteins to mimic the amino acid balance found naturally in animal products.

The popular Ezekiel 4:9 brand of bread products illustrates this principle. Based on a biblical command from God to the prophet Ezekiel, these bread products are made from a combination of wheat, barley, beans, lentils, millet, and spelt. Ezekiel was instructed to eat this bread for 390 days as a symbol of Israel's coming siege and exile, which would last for 390 years because of their idolatry. Sure enough, while none of these grains alone is a complete source of protein, when sprouted and combined they provide all nine essential amino acids. A similar technique is used to create viable plant-based protein powders, which often combine isolated pea and rice proteins to achieve a complete and relatively balanced amino acid profile.

But while sourcing the right concentrations of essential amino acids from plants is already a challenge, their absorption presents

---

278 Ibid.

another hurdle unique to vegan diets. Plant proteins are often more complex in structure and less accessible than animal proteins because they are often encased in cell walls. In addition, plants contain anti-nutrients—compounds that reduce the bioavailability of nutrients. Some compounds in legumes, grains, and seeds bind to proteins and inhibit digestion and assimilation. Digestive enzyme inhibitors, also common in these foods, further complicate the body's ability to break down and absorb amino acids. Fortunately, many of these antinutrients can be reduced or eliminated through soaking, sprouting, fermenting, or cooking—processes not required for animal proteins, which are naturally more absorbable and better tolerated.

Retinol. The folly of the crusade against animal fat becomes particularly evident when we consider that retinol—the only bioactive form of vitamin A—is derived exclusively from animal products and is essential for several physiological functions. As mentioned before, beta-carotene from foods such as carrots and sweet potatoes can be converted to retinol, but in much smaller amounts than when it is consumed directly.

Critical Minerals. Animal products are also rich in bioavailable minerals such as magnesium, copper, iodine, selenium, heme iron, and zinc. In contrast, plant sources often contain lower concentrations of these minerals, and anti-nutrients like phytates and oxalates can inhibit their absorption. Iodine deficiency is particularly common among those who rely solely on a plant-based diet, further highlighting the challenge of achieving adequate mineral intake without animal products.[279]

Animal Products and Iron

This raises an important question: if iron overload is a concern, wouldn't the abundant iron in meat and other animal products be problematic? Despite the apparent contradiction, it's important to recognize the difference between the iron found in nutrient-dense foods and that in synthetic supplements or iron-fortified products. Iron from nutrient-

---

279 Ibid.

dense sources, such as liver, is accompanied by essential cofactors like copper and retinol, which help the body properly regulate and metabolize it. In contrast, synthetic supplements and iron-fortified processed foods lack these supporting nutrients, making their iron more likely to contribute to imbalance and dysfunction. While it's important to monitor iron levels as a part of a comprehensive diagnostic routine, it's not necessary to avoid animal products for the sake of iron levels.

Omega-3 Fatty Acids. Finally, omega-3 fatty acids, particularly EPA and DHA, are critical for brain function, cardiovascular health, and reducing inflammation. These fatty acids are found almost exclusively in animal products such as fatty fish, cod liver oil, krill oil, and grass-fed beef. While plant foods such as flaxseeds and walnuts contain ALA, a precursor to EPA and DHA, the body's conversion efficiency is extremely low—typically less than 10 percent for EPA and less than 1 percent for DHA.[280] Although algae-based EPA and DHA supplements can provide a viable alternative for those on plant-based diets, they are far less potent and far more expensive than their animal-based counterparts.

The nutritional debate between animal- and plant-based food sources could fill volumes. Meat, especially red meat, and other animal products have long been criticized for their natural fats and cholesterol, both of which have historically been linked to heart disease. However, as we've previously explored, these concerns were a misplaced blind spot of the medical establishment, largely debunked by more rigorous science and reporting in recent years. When freed from these biases, the conversation shifts to a simple matter of nutrient density and availability.

Simply put, the lower nutrient density and bioavailability of plant-based foods often requires greater food intake, careful combination, and

---

280 In *Good Energy*, Casey Means points out that this inefficiency may stem from common nutrient deficiencies, as the enzymes responsible for this process require several B vitamins, vitamin C, zinc, and magnesium to function effectively, with 92 percent of the population deficient in at least one of these nutrients. Correcting these deficiencies, she suggests, may improve the conversion rate and make plant-based diets more viable.

supplementation to achieve the same nutritional profiles as animal-based diets.

For example, one hundred grams of protein can be obtained from an eight-ounce steak, a large glass of milk, and ten ounces of yogurt. To get the same from a vegan diet would require consuming over two pounds of cooked quinoa, twenty ounces of lentils, and 10.5 ounces of spinach—far beyond the caloric needs of most people.

No one would argue that modern societies are deficient in calories. But despite the energy density of our diets, most people remain starved for critical nutrients. If there's one thing animals are good at, it's concentrating these vital nutrients.

In conclusion, a healthy diet can take many forms, ranging from plant-centric to more animal-inclusive. The crucial takeaway, however, is that the omnivorous diet's inherent and unique ability to provide optimal nutrition across diverse climates, geographies, and economic circumstances underscores its place as a permissible and practical element of God's design for human flourishing.

A Biblical Approach to Animal Consumption

Now that we've explored some common critiques of animal consumption, it's time to summarize a biblical perspective on the matter. In short, the answer is neither rigidly anti-meat nor unconditionally pro-meat, but reflects humanity's unique and complex position in history.

First, we must acknowledge our special place in the hierarchy of creation, set above both plants and animals. This is evident in Scripture: God uniquely calls human beings by name, was incarnated as a human being, and has a special role for humanity in His redemptive plan. Yet, plants and animals occupy and animate the living space entrusted to human care. They are essential components of God's creative intent, and their existence and flourishing not only glorify God in themselves, but are fundamental for humanity's own existence and flourishing.

While plants were explicitly given to both humans and animals for food as an aspect of God's original creative will, the mention of animals for human food is conspicuously absent. As discussed earlier, this fact alone doesn't necessarily give us a definitive insight into God's plan for meat, since there is reasonable doubt as to whether it was actually forbidden or simply omitted. But a preponderance of the evidence suggests that meat was not a part of that original plan. Neither was a fallen humanity, however, yet that is our current state. It is only in the context of this fallen state that we find an explicit addition to mankind's original diet, where God says to Noah after the flood, "Into your hand [animals] are delivered. Every moving thing that lives shall be food for you. And as I gave you the green plants, I give you everything" (Gen. 9:2–3).

Barth emphasizes the distinction between the diet permitted to humans in their original, sinless state and the diet permitted in the fallen state. He suggests that while the consumption of animals may not have been a part of God's original intent and thus "stands under a caveat," it is nevertheless provided for a sinful humanity that God still graciously preserves against a hostile world.[281] According to Barth, we sin when we fail to recognize the caveat under which meat is provided as a gift from God for use in this present state of humanity. Thus, we should not presume to kill animals under our own authority as stewards of creation, but we should instead be aware of the qualified use of animals for which authority is provided by God. We kill and use animals ethically when we acknowledge this fact, and when, through this awareness, we surrender the animal to God, only to receive it from Him as something that satisfies our own needs and desires.[282]

Meat, therefore, is a gracious gift—not given reluctantly but generously provided for human flourishing. While Christians have sometimes been hesitant to embrace this provision, it is reaffirmed in the New Testament through Peter's vision of a sheet descending from heaven, filled with all kinds of animals. God's command to him—"Rise,

---

281 Barth, *Church Dogmatics*, 353.
282 Ibid., 355.

kill, and eat" (Acts 10:13)—not only emphasizes the spiritual inclusion of Gentiles and the fulfillment of the Mosaic dietary laws, but also implies the broad permissibility of animal consumption under the New Covenant.

Therefore, while abstaining from meat or other animal products is an acceptable personal choice, labeling it as unclean or unbiblical elevates human reason above divine intent. As Paul warns in 1 Timothy, the logic of man is often a false teacher.

> "[They] forbid marriage and require abstinence from foods that God created to be received with thanksgiving by those who believe and know the truth. For everything created by God is good, and nothing is to be rejected if it is received with thanksgiving." (1 Tim. 4:3–4)

He suggests that those who truly "know the truth" are characterized by their ability to see through worldly wisdom and instead receive the world as a gift to be enjoyed—sometimes in the form of a bacon-wrapped filet mignon.

And if anyone demonstrated this ability, it was Jesus himself, who was certainly not a vegan. In fact, there is ample evidence that Jesus ate animal flesh while on earth. As a faithful Jew, He partook of the Passover lamb each year.[283] He also miraculously multiplied fish for five thousand followers near the Sea of Galilee and presumably ate some himself, a miracle that would be rather odd for a God who doesn't approve of animal consumption.[284] We've already discussed that Jesus ate animal flesh on at least two occasions after His resurrection, demonstrating His physical presence by eating broiled fish in front of his disciples and by preparing a breakfast of bread and fish for His disciples by the Sea of Galilee.

If the author and perfecter of our faith considered a vegetarian diet to be ideal for a righteous life, shouldn't we expect Him to have

---

283 Mark 14:12–18 describes the Last Supper, which is understood by most historians to have been a Passover meal with Jesus and His disciples.

284 Luke 24:41–43

rebuked his flesh-eating followers for their pagan hedonism? Given His countercultural critiques, the widespread practice of eating meat would surely have warranted correction if it contradicted God's design. But Scripture offers no such rebuke.

Thus, we can confidently conclude that God intends for meat to be part of the human diet, consumed in gratitude and with an awareness of its divine provision.

Comparing Beef, Chicken, and Pork

Beef has long been criticized for its saturated-fat content, while chicken is often praised as a "lean, heart-healthy" choice. Pork, dubbed "the other white meat" yet biologically classed as red meat (and historically labeled "unclean" under Levitical law), often sits somewhere in between. How should we think about these three staples?

In short, none of these meats is inherently harmful, but with a catch: chicken and pork warrant much more caution than beef. Pigs and poultry are single-stomached, so the fats they eat become the fats we eat. Industrial diets—corn, soy, and other grain by-products—are rich in omega-6 PUFAs. Unable to convert these PUFAs into saturated fat, chickens and pigs deposit them intact. Consequently, conventional pork and chicken fat can have up to 20 percent omega-6 PUFA, while typical beef fat hovers around 2 percent.[285][286] Although these fats come from whole foods rather than ultra-processed oils, the dosage is anything but natural and may drive the same pro-inflammatory, fat-promoting metabolic signals associated with inflammatory oils.

---

285 L. Cortinas et al., "Fatty Acid Content in Chicken Thigh and Breast as Affected by Dietary Polyunsaturation Level," Poultry Science 83, no. 7 (July 2004): 1155–64, https://doi.org/10.1093/ps/83.7.1155.

286 Karola Gläser, Caspar Wenk, and Martin Scheeder, "Effect of Dietary Mono- and Polyunsaturated Fatty Acids on the Fatty Acid Composition of Pigs' Adipose Tissues," Archiv für Tierernährung 56 (2002): 51–65, https://doi.org/10.1080/00039420214178.

In short, beef is not the villain it's often made out to be. Why would God have provided Israel exclusively red meat if it was so bad? Chicken and pork, which are far less resilient, aren't inherently bad either but warrant serious caution when conventionally raised.

Conclusion

The belief that meat, especially red meat, is inherently harmful from every perspective is often unquestioned in popular culture. Whether criticized from theological, ethical, nutritional, or environmental angles, the anti-meat movement has embedded its ideas so deeply into society that they are often seen as beyond rational criticism. Robb Wolf aptly refers to these anti-meat sentiments as a modern "sacred cow." However, given how these views have repeatedly permeated Christian theology, it may be more fitting to compare them to a golden calf—an idol that distracts from obedience to God and risks unnecessary division within His kingdom.

A holistic theological and nutritional assessment of the consumption of meat and animal products should reassure the omnivorous Christian. There are, however, other indirect factors that could still affect the place of animals in a Christian diet.

The environmental impact of meat consumption deserves careful consideration, especially in light of the fact that our treatment of the environment is inherently theological and that the current cultural backlash against meat is largely motivated by concerns about its perceived environmental harm. For these reasons, the place of meat in a dietary paradigm that accounts for humanity's God-given role as stewards of the earth is left for the next chapter—and the conclusion may be surprising.

11

Steak and Stewardship (Envisioning a Biblical Food System)

*"Is it not enough for you to feed on the good
pasture, that you must tread down with
your feet the rest of your pasture; and to
drink of clear water, that you must muddy
the rest of the water with your feet?"*

— EZEKIEL 34:18

As we refine our nutritional paradigm, weaving together
theological and scientific insights into the spiritual and ethical
dimensions of our nourishment, it's important to revisit the way
of eating modeled in the Lord's Supper. Eucharistic eating reminds us to
perceive food as a manifestation of God's love and to seriously consider
whether our diets are consistent with the logic of God's design and
further His good purposes on earth. Food should invite us to consider
our neediness as creatures, reminding us that human beings are at the
center of a complex web of creation, and that only through our conscious
participation in and reconciliation with this creation can we come to
terms with our own nature.

In other words, our approach to food cannot be reduced to merely what, how, and when we eat, as if these choices exist in isolation. We must also acknowledge how food gets to our tables—how food systems contribute to a holistic understanding of nutrition.

Numerous important questions arise when considering this topic: Do these systems provide dignified work and fair wages? Do they support diverse cultural traditions? Do they yield healthy food in abundance? These are all worthy questions, for they all bear witness to the Logos of creation—the logic of God's good design.

The particular focus of this chapter, however, is on how food systems can help fulfill mankind's special role as *stewards of creation*. Through the lens of stewardship, we may discover that many other important aspects of ethical food production naturally fall into place.

In considering our stewardship of the earth, we inevitably encounter the controversial concept of environmentalism. Here, faithful Christians may find both common ground and points of divergence with mainstream environmental thought. While secular environmental movements can arise from a sincere desire to protect and preserve the beauty of creation, they often lack the guiding principle of worshiping God rather than nature. Indeed, by elevating the earth or the cosmos to almost divine status, these movements inadvertently reveal humanity's innate spiritual longing. But a distinctively Christian approach to stewardship recognizes that creation itself is not worthy of worship, but rather is meant to serve as a witness to the Creator and His goodness.

Consider, for example, the widespread personification of nature as "Mother Nature." While seemingly harmless, this concept often functions as a pagan idol. Like God, Mother Nature is portrayed as demanding worship and exacting judgment, but unlike the *real* God, she lacks benevolence toward humanity and is often characterized as a force opposed to human development. In this framework, natural disasters are seen as punitive responses to human ambition, while abortion, at least according to some radical progressive environmentalists, is effectively a sacramental offering in her service.[287]

When environmentalism takes on such idolatrous overtones, it's tempting to throw out the baby with the bathwater.

"Nature is not our mother," warns G. K. Chesterton. But he also offers a uniquely Christian perspective: "Nature is our sister. We can be proud of her beauty since we have the same father."[288]

If conservative Christians truly saw nature as their sibling, would they be proud of humanity's treatment of it?

Christians, of all people, should be the most likely to promote a nuanced form of environmental stewardship that is consistent with fundamental truths about the relationship between humanity and the rest of creation. As Joel Salatin says, we shouldn't go so far as to confuse "creation worship" with "Creator worship." While radical hippie environmentalists may idolize nature, Christian stewardship calls for an orderly care of creation that honors and points back to its Creator. By examining how we manage the resources entrusted to us, we can not only complete our paradigm for nutrition, but also channel our need for food into a more robust and deeply embodied expression of faith.

First, it's important to recognize two fundamental principles of biblical environmental stewardship.

The Principles of Biblical Environmental Stewardship

Human Flourishing

The fact that creation exists out of the abundance of God's love and for the purpose of pleasing Him leads us to conclude that we should adore it as much as He does. But while all of creation is precious, human

---

287 Population reduction through abortion access has been tied to radical environmentalism since the mid-twentieth century, reaching an extreme in Ginette Paris's work, *The Sacrament of Abortion*, which describes abortion as a sacrifice to the earth goddess.

288 G. K. Chesterton, *Orthodoxy* (New York: Dodd, Mead & Company, 1908).

beings—made in God's image—occupy a uniquely exalted place within it.

In the Sermon on the Mount, Jesus teaches,

"Look at the birds of the air: they neither sow nor reap nor gather into barns, and yet your heavenly Father feeds them. Are you not of more value than they? ... Consider the lilies of the field, how they grow: they neither toil nor spin, yet I tell you, even Solomon in all his glory was not arrayed like one of these. But if God so clothes the grass of the field, which today is alive and tomorrow is thrown into the oven, will he not much more clothe you, O you of little faith?" (Matt. 6:26, 28–30)

According to Jesus, not even the great King Solomon could surpass the splendor of a single lily. But while the earth will eventually be destroyed, believers will continue to live in a personal relationship with their Creator. In this way, Jesus acknowledges humanity's supremacy over creation without neglecting to cherish the beauty of the world He created.

This implies that God's creation is designed for human flourishing, a theme that echoes what many call God's "cultural mandate," described in Genesis 1:28:

And God blessed them. And God said to them, "Be fruitful and multiply and fill the earth and subdue it, and have dominion over the fish of the sea and over the birds of the heavens and over every living thing that moves on the earth."

The commands to "be fruitful," "multiply," and "fill the earth" are inseparable.

God entrusts resources—air, water, trees, minerals, and animals—to humanity, not merely for their preservation, but also for their responsible and imaginative use in the name of human progress and flourishing.

If there's any doubt that this is God's intention, we should recall that while the story of mankind begins with a farmer and his wife in an untended garden, it culminates in the New Jerusalem—a grand city adorned with an array of natural resources, precisely arranged as if crafted by a divine artisan. This majestic city is described in the Book of Revelation:

> "The wall was built of jasper, while the city was pure gold, like clear glass. The foundations of the wall of the city were adorned with every kind of jewel … And the twelve gates were twelve pearls, each of the gates made of a single pearl, and the street of the city was pure gold, like transparent glass." (Rev. 21:18–21)

Stewardship, then, isn't just about preserving the earth as if it were untouched by humanity; rather, the earth, while beautiful in its pristine state, is to bear the imprint of humanity's labor and creativity, wisely used in service of our own flourishing.

Dominion Balanced with Care

This purposeful stewardship of the earth is to be carried out according to a dual mandate from God: to balance our *authority* over the earth with our duty to *care* for it.

The first half of this mandate, authority, comes from God's instruction to "subdue" the earth and "have dominion" over "every living thing that moves on the earth" (Gen. 1:28). These strong verbs indicate a delegation of divine authority that gives humanity not only the right but also the responsibility to exercise it. Fruitful stewardship requires this kind of dominion, calling us to be bold, thoughtful, and skillful in managing the earth's plants, animals, and resources.[289]

This authority, however, must be balanced by our responsibility to care for creation. The first tasks given to Adam were to "dress" and "keep" the Garden of Eden (Gen. 2:15).[290] The key verb "keep" implies preserving, guarding, and protecting from harm, all concepts that evoke

---

289 *Cambridge Bible for Schools and Colleges,* Cambridge: Cambridge University Press, 1893.

290 Just because these activities were given only to one man at one time in history doesn't mean that we should neglect their applicability today. The anthropological value of this creation account implies that these duties are tied to our human nature, in general.

the modern idea of environmental conservation—the responsible care of the land, water, air, plant and animal life, and climate.

In balancing our authority over the earth with its care, God suggests that there is both wisdom and goodness in His designs—that humanity is to both adore and advance *His* logic if we are ultimately to be fruitful in our stewardship.

Our fallen nature often tempts us to isolate virtues and take them to extremes. But our dominion doesn't allow us to pillage and rape the earth any more than our care allows us to leave it untouched. Neither half of this dual mandate can be separated from the other, for God delights in people reaping the fruits of His creation while ensuring that it remains viable for use by the next generation.

Attributes of a Biblical Food System

A nutrition paradigm, if it is to be Christian in any sense, must acknowledge the inescapable fact that food production is one of the primary ways in which humans interact with the earth and its resources. It is this recognition that brings environmental stewardship into the equation.

The central question, then, is how to promote food systems that are compatible with these basic principles of biblical stewardship. What characteristics must a food system have to promote human flourishing while balancing our God-given authority over creation with our obligation to care for it?

In two words, such a food system must be *fruitful* and *sustainable*. It should be productive enough to reflect God's abundant provision, and it should be maintainable over the long run.

But while we have arguably been pretty good at creating a fruitful, productive food system—at least in terms of unprecedented amounts of food—there's no doubt that we've done so at the expense of our ability to sustain it. Today's food systems are defined less by their sustainability than by their exploitation—systems that deplete finite resources and demand ever-increasing inputs to simply sustain production. Exploitative systems prioritize short-term abundance at the expense of long-term viability by compromising the very inputs on which they depend.

Our rapidly depleting soil illustrates the dangers of exploitative agriculture, for just as humanity was created from the soil, our fate is intimately tied to its health. Industrial farming practices, such as heavy use of pesticides and herbicides combined with aggressive tillage, strip fertile soil of its life-sustaining properties, turning it into mere dirt. This lifeless dirt is then artificially enriched with synthetic fertilizers to maintain crop yields. But while this approach has led to increased productivity, it has come at a steep cost. As topsoil declines, so does its productivity, forcing farmers to double down on their exploitative methods just to maintain yields, and perpetuating a vicious cycle of degradation and diminished returns.

Another consequence of degraded soil is its inability to retain water effectively. Unlike healthy, spongy soil, lifeless dirt repels water. Is it a mere coincidence that the American Midwest has been plagued by heavy water runoff and flash flooding in recent years?

This runoff not only causes erosion and accelerates the land degradation caused by industrial monoculture farming, but it also pollutes critical waterways. Nitrogen and phosphorus from synthetic fertilizers are washed into rivers and lakes, triggering harmful algal blooms that deplete oxygen, kill aquatic life, and create vast hypoxic zones. Industrial farming practices have polluted the Mississippi River to the point that a dead zone the size of New Jersey has formed in the Gulf of America (formerly known as the Gulf of Mexico), and its expansion is accelerating with increased fertilizer use and water runoff.

Concentrated animal feeding operations (CAFOs) exacerbate the problem of water pollution. Manure runoff not only adds nitrogen and phosphorus to the water, further contributing to harmful algal blooms, but it also injects a cocktail of harmful pathogens such as bacteria (E. coli and salmonella), viruses, and parasites, and unwanted pharmaceuticals such antibiotics and hormones. These contaminants not only harm aquatic life or contribute to antibiotic resistance, but they can also affect our drinking water.

Finally, while concerns about soil and water health are pressing, many are focusing on the long-term effects of greenhouse gas emissions from agriculture. While belching cows get a lot of flak for their contribution to methane emissions—a natural byproduct of digestion—the real problem, as we'll explore, lies in exploitative farming practices.

Consider the amazing fact that the Earth contains 3,170 gigatons of carbon, and about 80 percent of it is stored in the form of soil. By plundering our topsoil, we are releasing massive amounts of this carbon into the atmosphere, where it can remain for thousands of years. The dirt that's left has to be fertilized with something, and that's where fossil fuels add to the gaseous pollution. To make ammonia (NH_3) fertilizers, nitrogen is sucked out of the air and combined with hydrogen from natural gas, a very energy-intensive process that releases CO_2 into the atmosphere as a byproduct of the hydrogen separation process. These synthetic fertilizers then create a double whammy of greenhouse gases when they are converted by the soil into nitrous oxide (N_2O), which has nearly 300 times the potential warming effect of carbon dioxide.

Sir Albert Howard, the "father of modern organic agriculture," warned that every generation faces the temptation to exploit the natural resources created over millennia and convert them into immediate financial gain. By failing to adopt a stewardship mindset, recent generations have turned healthy soil into cash crops that do little more than fuel our cars and make us fatter, sicker, and more depressed. When we consider the results of this cash-out, is it really a bargain?

When we grow food according to God's design, we enrich the soil instead of depleting it, protect waterways instead of polluting them, and keep carbon where it belongs. This is what a truly fruitful and sustainable food system looks like.

In the previous chapter, we explored the inclusion of animal products, especially meat, in the Christian paradigm for nutrition, addressing theological, ethical, and health considerations. However, these discussions often serve as a distraction from the real controversy: the environmental impact of meat.

With plant-based marketing dominating the narrative, it seems heretical to Mother Nature to suggest ditching veggie burgers for environmental reasons. Yet, there is no such thing as an ecosystem without animals, and so we should come to terms with the fact that God's design for sustainability requires our thoughtful participation in the ecosystems He has created.

To illustrate this point, let us briefly address some popular claims against the use of animals in food systems, focusing primarily on cows and other ruminants.

Addressing Environmental Claims Against Meat Production

"Meat Production is a Drain on Resources"

The SDA Church's beef with beef is multifaceted, but Ellen White articulated a point that plant-pushers have been regurgitating for generations: meat production is an inefficient use of resources. According to White,

> "Those who eat flesh are but eating grains and vegetables at second hand; for the animal receives from these things the nutrition that produces growth. The life that was in the grains and vegetables passes into the eater. We receive it by eating the flesh of the animal. How much better to get it direct, by eating the food that God provided for our use!"[291]

What if, following White's lead, the land currently used to grow feed for livestock were instead used to produce crops for direct human consumption, bypassing livestock as the "middlemen?" How much of our resources do these middlemen divert, anyway? Furthermore, to what extent are we inadvertently supporting exploitative monocrop farming practices to produce livestock feed?

There are many relevant considerations related to the use of resources in meat production, but they tend to boil down to one

---

291 White, *The Ministry of Healing.*

fundamental question: are livestock merely on our plates, or are they eating at our tables?[292]

If White were still with us, she might highlight popular statistics that seem to favor the conclusion that livestock are an inefficient waste of resources. For example, some people claim that it takes 12 to 20 pounds of feed to produce just one pound of beef, or that one acre of land can produce 50,000 pounds of tomatoes but only 250 pounds of beef.[293] At first glance, these numbers seem damning. How could a sustainable food system designed to feed a growing population justify such apparent inefficiency?

But despite the surface logic of these claims, they overlook critical points. Livestock, as we'll briefly explore, may not be as inefficient or wasteful as superficial comparisons suggest.

When it comes to feed, no one would dispute the fact that livestock consume more total weight than they produce in meat or dairy products. But to truly evaluate the question of whether livestock are on our plates or eating at our tables, it's important to compare the nutrient density of what they eat with what they produce.

Starting with inputs, let's recognize that ruminants were never meant to share the same menu as humans. Because humans have only one stomach, we cannot break down the cellulose in grass and other fibrous plants; these substances would be useless or even harmful to us. Ruminants, on the other hand, have specialized digestive systems that can extract nutrients from this indigestible plant matter and convert it into high-quality protein and essential nutrients that humans can easily absorb.

---

292 This phrase is attributed to Anne Mottet et al., "Livestock: On Our Plates or Eating at Our Table? A New Analysis of the Feed/Food Debate," *Global Food Security* 14 (September 2017): 1–8.

293 Paul R. Ehrlich and Anne H. Ehrlich, *Population, Resources, Environment* (San Francisco: W. H. Freeman, 1970). Ehrlich famously predicted that by the 1980s hundreds of millions of people would starve to death due to the inability of the planet to sustain such a rapidly growing human population.

That said, it is true that most ruminant livestock today are not exclusively grass-fed, often spending the last few months of their lives feeding on grains that are diverted from potentially feeding humans directly.[294] But even within the current industrial system, the extent to which livestock consume human-edible food is vastly overstated.

A comprehensive 2017 analysis found that 86 percent of the world's current livestock feed is not fit for human consumption. Most of the feed is grass and leaves (46 percent), stalks and other fibrous plant residues (19 percent), and fodder crops (8 percent).[295] Only a measly 14 percent of livestock feed comes from human-edible crops like corn, soybeans, and wheat, often subsidized by taxpayers and funneled into industrial feedlots.

Even in these grain-based systems, livestock still produce more high-quality protein (in the form of milk or meat) than they consume from human-edible sources—about 67 percent more, according to the same study.[296] But even this fact fails to capture their full glory, which goes beyond their ability to provide high-quality protein, natural fats, and other concentrated nutrients. They also enhance our lives by providing materials for other everyday products, such as leather seats and tennis racket strings. Even their poop is useful, contributing to healthy soils and vibrant ecosystems.

So if ruminants are middlemen at all, they are uniquely charitable ones, taking no cut of the profits but instead multiplying the benefits for the end consumer. As sustainable food advocate Diana Rodgers puts it, ruminants don't just use nutrients—they *upcycle* them, turning otherwise unusable resources into valuable outputs.[297]

---

294 "Grass-fed" is a misleading term, as regulations on its use are varied and generally unclear. Typically, both grass-fed and conventional cattle graze on grass for most of their lives and are switched to a grain-based feedlot diet to speed up weight gain prior to being slaughtered. "Grass-finished" cattle, on the other hand, are never introduced to grain and exclusively graze on grass.

295 Anne Mottet et al., "Livestock: On Our Plates or Eating at Our Table?".

296 Ibid.

297 Diana Rodgers and Robb Wolf, *Sacred Cow: The Case for (Better) Meat* (New York: BenBella Books, 2020), 152.

This point cannot be overstated: the unique glory of ruminants is their capacity to transform what is inedible to humans into nutrient-dense food.

The question of responsible land use remains, however. Couldn't the land that produces these grasses be used to grow edible crops instead?

Critics point out that one acre of land can produce 50,000 pounds of tomatoes, 53,000 pounds of potatoes, or 30,000 pounds of carrots, but only about 250 pounds of beef. Again, on the surface, this seems like an open-and-shut case against livestock.

However, this comparison suffers from two major flaws.

First, while tomatoes, potatoes, and carrots may yield more weight per acre, they fall far short of beef in terms of nutrient density. For example, it takes about 29 pounds of tomatoes, 13 pounds of potatoes, or 29 pounds of carrots to match the protein content of just one pound of beef. The disparity becomes even more pronounced when comparing essential amino acids such as leucine, which are critical for muscle synthesis and overall health. Adjusting the comparison to reflect nutrient density rather than mere weight significantly narrows the apparent disparity. However, even with these adjustments, livestock undeniably require more land than plant-based food sources, a reality critics often exaggerate but need not dismiss entirely.

This disparity, however, is reframed when we account for the actual type and availability of land. Just as it's misleading to equate tomatoes and beef based solely on weight, it's equally misguided to treat fertile cropland and marginal pastureland as interchangeable. Equating these two types of land is akin to comparing prime Malibu real estate with Skid Row.

Highly fertile and productive cropland, which produces thousands of pounds of vegetables, constitutes only a small fraction of the world's agricultural land—about one-third. The remaining two-thirds of agricultural land consists largely of pastureland, which is unsuitable for growing crops but is ideal for growing native grasses that support ruminants such as cattle.[298] Livestock grazing transforms these otherwise unproductive lands into nutrient-rich food, while improving soil fertility, water retention and biodiversity.

Thus, when we consider the total amount of nutrients that could be generated across all agricultural land—including both cropland and grazing land—the case for ruminants as an essential part of sustainable food systems becomes far more compelling.

Ruminants, therefore, should be fully absolved of the perception that they are a waste of food resources. However, if there is any validity to the claim that animal products are inefficient middlemen, the primary culprits are not cattle but rather chickens and pigs. Unlike ruminants— which can thrive on marginal land by consuming forage inedible to humans and, even in industrial farming systems, spend a significant portion of their lives grazing—chickens and pigs are typically raised exclusively on grains and crops grown on cropland that could otherwise produce food for direct human consumption.

These animals are indeed eating at our tables today, but that hasn't always been the case. Historically, they played a crucial role in food security and sanitation by converting food scraps, agricultural byproducts, and even human waste into valuable nutrient sources.

Chickens, for example, can thrive on an eclectic diet that includes vegetable peels, stale bread, worms, grubs, leafy plants, and seeds. Similarly, pigs are nature's consummate scavengers, capable of living off the roots, tubers, bugs, mushrooms, nuts, and fruits they forage. This adaptability has historically allowed them to complement agricultural systems rather than compete with humans for resources.

Today, however, industrial poultry and pork production relies heavily on grain-based feedlots, fueled by cheap oil (for synthetic fertilizers) and taxpayer subsidies. This dependence creates a precarious system that relies on political stability and finite fossil fuel reserves rather than the sun, the regenerative foundation of sustainable agriculture.

---

298 "Livestock on Grazing Lands," in *Livestock & the Environment: Meeting the Challenge* (FAO), accessed September 21, 2023, https://www.fao.org/3/x5304e/x5304e03.htm.

Under the current system, these animals are not exactly models of stewardship. But in a reimagined food system aligned with God's sun-powered design, every animal would have a place to fruitfully and sustainably express its glory. In such a system, cattle, sheep, and goats would graze on grass, enriching the soil as they go; chickens would eat kitchen scraps or follow larger livestock, pecking at grubs in the churned-up soil; and pigs would forage in forests, turning otherwise inedible materials into nutrient-dense food.

While this vision may sound utopian in light of our modern experience, it has already been proven feasible on a larger scale, as we'll discuss later. Animals, when thoughtfully integrated, don't drain resources—they unlock nutrients inaccessible to humans, increasing the sustainability and productivity of the land.

In short, from both a land and feed perspective, the business case for beef looks a whole lot better when we realize that humans can't eat grass, but we *can* eat cows. Why not let them turn that grass into nutrient-rich ribeye?

"But Belching Cows are Bad for the Climate"

In addition to being criticized as a drain on resources, ruminant livestock are frequently blamed as a major contributor to climate change. This is because their unique digestive systems cause them to belch methane (CH_4), a carbon-based greenhouse gas about 30 times as potent as carbon dioxide. According to the US Environmental Protection Agency, methane emissions from livestock account for about 2–3 percent of total US greenhouse gas emissions across all sectors.[299] But while 2 percent may sound insignificant, critics argue that even small percentages add up to alarming numbers when scaled globally. Indeed, it is estimated

---

299 "Agriculture and Aquaculture: Food for Thought," US EPA, February 27, 2023, https://www.epa.gov/snep/agriculture-and-aquaculture-food-thought; "Inventory of U.S. Greenhouse Gas Emissions and Sinks: 1990-2021," US EPA, February 14, 2024, https://www.epa.gov/ghgemissions/inventory-us-greenhouse-gas-emissions-and-sinks-1990-2021.

that the roughly one and a half billion cattle on the planet collectively emit a staggering 150 billion pounds of methane annually.

However, this narrative about ruminants and methane emissions is udderly misleading (pun intended) and ignores critical context.

First, it is important to recognize that North America was inhabited by large numbers of ruminants long before the term "global warming" was ever coined. Bison, elk, deer, and other herbivores collectively emitted methane levels estimated to be about 82 percent of current emissions from both wild and farmed ruminants.[300] While the global population of domesticated ruminants has tripled over the past century,[301] this increase has been largely offset by the decline of wild ruminants due to habitat loss, hunting, and human encroachment. Therefore, it's safe to say that while total ruminant emissions may have increased in the industrial era, they cannot account for the doubling of atmospheric methane levels over the past 200 years.

The real drivers of rising methane levels are fossil fuels and rice production. A NASA analysis attributes annual increases of about 17 teragrams of methane to the fossil fuel industry and 12 teragrams to rice production, with a reduction of four teragrams due to fewer fires.[302] Together, these sources fully explain the 25 teragrams of annual increase in atmospheric methane. Yet rice, a staple food for billions of people, escapes the same scrutiny as livestock. Why aren't there calls to eliminate rice paddies if methane emissions are a major problem?

The bigger issue with this logic, however, is the flawed comparison itself: the 2–3 percent of greenhouse gas emissions attributed to livestock shouldn't even be on the same graph as fossil fuel emissions. Methane from livestock is part of the biogenic carbon cycle—a regenerative, closed-loop system designed by God—whereas fossil fuel emissions

300 Alexander N. Hristov, "Historic, Pre-European Settlement, and Present-Day Contribution of Wild Ruminants to Enteric Methane Emissions in the United States," *Journal of Animal Science* 90, no. 4 (April 2012): 1371–75.

301 Statista, "Global Cattle Population from 1990 to 2022," Last modified 2022. https://www.statista.com/statistics/263979/global-cattle-population-since-1990/.

302 Carol Rasmussen, "NASA-led Study Solves a Methane Puzzle," *Climate Change: Vital Signs of the Planet*, June 13, 2018.

represent a one-way, extractive process that adds "new" carbon to the atmosphere. By conflating these fundamentally different systems, critics fail to acknowledge that animal methane operates within a sustainable, natural cycle, while fossil fuel emissions exacerbate the climate crisis by introducing carbon that has been locked away for millennia.

The methane emitted by ruminants remains in the atmosphere for about ten years before breaking down into water and carbon dioxide. This CO_2 is then absorbed by plants through photosynthesis, transformed back into plant matter, and consumed again by ruminants, perpetuating the cycle. Ruminants don't introduce new carbon to the atmosphere; they simply recycle the same carbon atoms over and over again. As Ecclesiastes reminds us, "What has been is what will be, and what has been done is what will be done, and there is nothing new under the sun" (Eccl. 1:9). It doesn't matter how much cows and goats belch; the net carbon emissions from ruminants are effectively zero.

In contrast to the cyclical carbon emissions of ruminants, fossil fuels release carbon that has been sequestered underground for millions of years, adding new carbon to the atmosphere. This distinction is critical: while carbon emissions are a legitimate concern, it is the introduction of this new carbon from fossil fuels that exacerbates the problem—not the recycled carbon emitted by ruminants.

To address the growing levels of atmospheric carbon, many have proposed technological solutions, such as carbon capture systems that condense CO_2 into solid forms for storage or reuse. These systems often involve large fans that draw air through chemical filters that absorb carbon, which must then be released, cleaned, compressed, and stored. While intriguing, these technologies are inherently energy-intensive, costly, and difficult to scale to meaningful levels.

But the idea of carbon capture is far from novel. In fact, God invented free, scalable carbon capture technology when He created plants, especially perennials.

Returning to the simplified carbon cycle, plants absorb CO_2 from the air and store it as plant matter, making them natural carbon sinks. However, there's a significant difference between the carbon sequestration abilities of *annuals*—plants that must be replanted each year—and *perennials*—plants that survive for several growing seasons, often dying back during the winter but regrowing in the spring. Annuals, such as corn, wheat, soybeans, and tomatoes, have shallow root systems and store their energy in seeds, often taking more energy from the soil than they give back. On top of this, because they must be replanted and harvested each year, the soil is often tilled and broken up by large combines, further degrading it. Perennials, like grass, on the other hand, store their energy underground in deep, complex root structures that build healthy, stable, and resilient soil year after year without the need for replanting.

Ruminants are an integral part of this system. Grazing animals such as cattle, sheep, and goats "self-harvest" perennial grasses, consuming some nutrients and returning the rest as manure, which is trampled into the soil to fertilize new growth. This natural process aerates the soil, improves fertility, and contributes to the formation of robust grasslands. In addition, ruminants can transport nutrients uphill through grazing, stabilizing slopes and enriching valleys as rain distributes the nutrients.

This regenerative effect is multiplied when robust grasslands influence local weather patterns, attracting more consistent rainfall to the area. Healthy soil acts like a sponge—the opposite of the hydrophobic dirt created by conventional farming practices. This means that it can better retain water and promote more consistent plant growth, which increases local humidity and encourages cloud formation and more consistent rainfall. Remarkably, this self-sustaining system can thrive year after year, as long as large herbivores are present to graze on the grass, completing the cycle.

Far from being a threat to the climate, well-managed livestock can actively maintain it by restoring healthy ecosystems. By improving water cycles, increasing biodiversity, and building carbon-rich soils, ruminants contribute to a massive carbon sink.

Agricultural practices that mimic natural patterns—commonly known as "regenerative agriculture"—leverage these benefits to promote sustainability. A prime example is multi-species pasture rotation, which imitates the natural movement of wild herbivores once guided by predators. Unlike the stagnant, overgrazed plots of conventional systems, rotational grazing ensures animals consume only the tops of grasses, preserving root systems and allowing the land to rest and rejuvenate. Their dung and urine naturally fertilize the soil, accelerating recovery and boosting productivity. This dynamic process showcases how livestock, when thoughtfully managed, can transform degraded lands into thriving ecosystems.

Regenerative agriculture is arguably the most effective carbon sequestration technology available, and there are plenty of case studies to prove it. To demonstrate the effectiveness of these methods, Michigan State University published a life cycle analysis of pasture-raised beef from White Oak Pastures, a regenerative farm in Georgia. Amazingly, the analysis found that the farm's holistically managed pastures *returned* 3.5 kilograms of CO_2 to the soil for every kilogram of beef produced, all while turning a healthy profit.[303]

For comparison, Impossible Meat, a leading producer of "eco-friendly," plant-based "meat," commissioned the same researchers to analyze the carbon footprint of its products. The study found that for every kilogram of fake meat produced, 3.5 kilograms of CO_2 were *emitted* from the ground—precisely the opposite of regenerative beef.[304] As Robb Wolf wryly observes, eating a White Oak Pastures burger may be the best way to offset the emissions of a supposedly "green" fake meat burger.

Better yet, White Oak Pastures was, until recently, a farm that relied on conventional, exploitative practices, offering a compelling testimony that highlights the shortcomings of conventional farming while providing a roadmap for better, regenerative practices:

"Fewer than 20 years ago, White Oak Pastures had evolved into a conventionally run commodity cattle farm. We employed all of the industrial tools that science had developed to take the

---

303 White Oak Pastures Team, "Regenerative Agriculture Vs. Fake Meat," *White Oak Pastures Blog*, accessed September 4, 2024, https://blog.whiteoakpastures.com/blog/grassfed-beef-vs-fake-meat.

304 "Impossible Burger Environmental Life Cycle Assessment 2019," accessed September 4, 2024, https://impossiblefoods.com/sustainable-food/burger-life-cycle-assessment-2019.

costs out of farming, including pesticides, chemical fertilizers, hormones, and antibiotics. Even while using these artificial crutches, our family never ceased to believe that we were being good stewards of our land. We were completely oblivious to the grave consequences that can result from fighting against nature. We were unwittingly steering our family heritage in a direction that was not environmentally sustainable ... Today, we are raising cattle, sheep, goats, hogs, poultry, and rabbits using the same methods ... used a century-and-a-half ago. We proactively support nature's food chain, using only sun, soil, and rain to grow sweet grasses for our animals to eat. Using Regenerative Land Management, we rotate complementary animal species side-by-side through our pastures. The cows graze the grass, the sheep and goats eat the weeds and shrubs, and the chickens peck at the grubs and insects. All species naturally fertilize the land, and our soil is again a living organic medium that teems with life."[305]

Although the testimony does not explicitly identify the farm as Christian, its practices reflect a profoundly biblical vision of stewardship. In producing food for his community and supporting his family, the owner of this farm paints a mural of God's wisdom, grace, and abundance. His model combines dominion and care in a way that honors the land and animals entrusted to him, allowing each to express its unique glory according to God's design—all while pulling carbon out of the atmosphere and putting it in the ground.

This regenerative model stands in stark contrast to the exploitative practices that dominate most farms today. While concerns about ruminant emissions are largely exaggerated, the destructive methods of industrial animal agriculture cannot be excused or upheld. The goal is not merely to defend the status quo, but to restore agricultural systems that align with God's cyclical, sun-powered design for sustainable stewardship. What seems innovative in regenerative farming is, in fact,

---

305 "Land Regeneration," White Oak Pastures, accessed September 4, 2024, https://whiteoakpastures.com/pages/environmental-sustainability.

a revival of ancient practices—practices that work in harmony with creation rather than against it.

"A Regenerative Food System is Far too Labor Intensive"

Finally, one more criticism often leveled against this fruitful and sustainable food system is that it relies too heavily on human and animal labor.

There is some truth to this concern, as we mentioned in Chapter Three when discussing the supposed societal accomplishment of reducing the portion of the population involved in food production. Shifting from conventional to animal-based, regenerative practices would indeed require more, smaller farms and more people stepping away from socially prestigious, white-collar jobs to engage in work often stereotyped as suitable only for "hicks" or migrant laborers.

But would it really be a disaster to reduce the labor force devoted to treating chronic diseases, developing pharmaceuticals, designing more effective herbicides, or lobbying for the processed food industry if the alternative was a thriving small-scale agricultural system that addressed these issues with real food? A shift to such a system could fundamentally reshape how we approach food production and health, offering solutions grounded in nutrient-dense, sustainably produced food rather than reactive measures to manage the consequences of industrial farming.

Of course, the current state of industrial farming makes it easy to understand why many are repulsed by the idea of agricultural work. Few would willingly choose a career that involves spraying deadly chemicals, debeaking chickens, collecting dead animals in a hazmat suit, or, in the worst cases, falling into a manure lagoon. Beyond these grim realities, modern industrial farming imposes enormous stress on those who manage it. Annual dependence on expensive external inputs—seeds, feeds, synthetic fertilizers, pesticides, and industrial machinery—places a significant financial burden on farmers each season. These upfront costs translate into massive debt and substantial risk, with profitability often hinging on volatile commodity prices and the unpredictability of the harvest. Given these financial burdens, is it any wonder that farmers have significantly higher rates of anxiety, depression, and suicide than the rest of the population?[306]

In contrast, multi-species pasture rotation methods require minimal inputs. These systems thrive with little more than native perennial grasses, temporary fencing, tarps, and basic tools like pliers. Joel Salatin relates the story of Gordon Hazard, an iconic rancher who boasted that he could manage three thousand steers with nothing more than a pickup truck. When times got tough, Salatin says, he could ditch the truck.

The simplicity and resilience of regenerative methods means lower risk and liberation from costly externalities. Moreover, these approaches create diversified revenue streams, making them more sustainable and less stressful for farmers. And the scalable nature of these methods means that even families without commercial farming ambitions can experiment with ways to make their land more fruitful.

After the Fall, God said to Adam,

"Cursed is the ground because of you; in pain you shall eat of it all the days of your life; thorns and thistles it shall bring forth for you; and you shall eat the plants of the field. By the sweat of your face you shall eat bread till you return to the ground. (Gen. 3:17–19)

This verse describes the first time that producing food became a toil, but it would be a mistake to see this labor as merely punishment. Read in the light of God's mercy and abundant provision, we can draw a different conclusion: hard work is an essential part of interacting with a fallen world. Work that strives toward God's design for life can be deeply

---

306 A. Bjornestad, C. Cuthbertson, and J. Hendricks, 2021, "An Analysis of Suicide Risk Factors among Farmers in the Midwestern United States," *International Journal of Environmental Research and Public Health* 18: 3563.

dignifying and sanctifying, especially when it yields beauty, profitability, and a testimony to God's goodness and abundance.

We won't all become regenerative ranchers, but we should consider how we can encourage and participate in this life-giving, restorative work—work that offers a picture of the flourishing that God intends for creation, and stands in stark contrast to the exploitation, debt, and stress of the industrial food system we have inherited.

A Better Way

Stewardship is a theme woven throughout the Christian life as we seek to manage what God has entrusted to us—our bodies, finances, land, and animals—in a way that honors Him. We've already explored this theme in the context of health, recognizing that the strength we cultivate through our eating habits has consequences beyond a simple number on the scale, equipping us to do the works God has prepared for us. In this chapter, we've broadened the focus to include our role as stewards of creation as a whole. In doing so, we've found that just as plants and animals have distinct roles in our diet, a biblical food system is both fruitful and sustainable to the extent that it embraces and magnifies their unique glories as well.

Whether we realize it or not, we all play an active role in shaping the food system. The real question is how we can take a more intentional, participatory role as members in a God-honoring food system. The answers are many: we can buy directly from farms that produce food in harmony with God's design; challenge the industrial egg industry by raising backyard chickens to turn food scraps into nutrient-dense eggs; and avoid highly processed foods that prop up industrial monoculture farming.

In other words, we can ask, "Is the food I'm eating helping to build soil or depleting it?" If the answer tends toward the former, it's likely that this food is also nourishing healthy bodies, strengthening communities, and serving as a tangible reflection of God's grand design for human flourishing as a byproduct.

Conclusion

*"To the world, which belongs to those with
tongues to taste it: Na Zdrovie! To God Who gives
the world to those with tongues: Er lebe hoch!
And to the vast paradox by which the One enjoys
the other: Bottoms up! Creation deserves the
most resounding slap we can give it... He fathers
forth whose beauty is past change. Praise Him!"*

— ROBERT FARRAR CAPON, THE SUPPER OF THE LAMB

As we conclude, it's fitting to reflect again on David's powerful invitation in Psalm 34:8: "Taste and see that the Lord is good." This is a call for more than just spiritual reflection; it invites us into a deeply embodied and sensory encounter with God's goodness. Of all our senses, taste is perhaps the most intimate and visceral. We can observe or listen to something from a distance, but to taste is to bring it into ourselves, to make it part of who we are. Just as we savor the food that nourishes our physical bodies, we are called to "taste" and experience God's sustaining presence in every area of life—to see how God satisfies all of our hungers. It's as if David is extending his hand to offer us something new, promising, "If you try it, you'll like it."

Our constant need for food is perhaps the single most tangible manifestation of our total dependence on God. The way we respond to this physical necessity has profound implications—not just for our physical health but for our spiritual lives as well. Sadly, many people, including Christians, fail to see this connection, and most nutrition paradigms lack a proper foundation that acknowledges the Creator's design for both body and soul. The obvious question, then, is how we can start to satisfy *all* our hungers and glorify God through a uniquely Christian approach to nutrition.

The answer, as this book has sought to demonstrate, can only be found in Christ: the Redeemed Body, the Bread of Life, and the Divine Physician. In other words, Jesus is the perfect compass pointing to God's design for nutrition.

To begin, we must recognize and appreciate that the human person—the one who eats—is a whole, a psychosomatic union of body, soul, and spirit. Christians have long been tempted to minimize the significance of the body, focusing instead on the spiritual or intellectual aspects of faith. But God never intended this divide. Looking back at our origin story, we see that the body is a visible manifestation of the otherwise invisible aspects of our personhood, designed to plainly reveal our nature as beings created in His image.

Having established this high view of the body, we must consider what constitutes a body in the first place. Contemplating the duality of our form and material reveals two truths: on the one hand, we cannot be reduced to the sum of our parts; on the other hand, we are constantly in flux, integrated with the world around us, always both feeding on and feeding the rest of creation. These complementary aspects of our nature highlight the richness of God's design and invite us to the profound possibility of joining ourselves to Christ through participation in His bride, the Church—a mystical reality made practical and intuitive through food.

Simply put, Jesus redeems the body by putting better food and drink in it. He says, "For my flesh is true food, and my blood is true drink," and also declares, "Whoever comes to me shall not hunger, and whoever believes in me shall never thirst" (Jn. 6:55; 35). As our perfect High Priest, Jesus takes the simple elements of bread and wine and uses them to give new life to believers.

Food takes on profound meaning when understood in this light. By eating Eucharistically, we elevate what might otherwise be a mundane necessity—or even a hedonistic indulgence—into a means of grace. This practice teaches us to faithfully receive God's gift of life and acknowledge Him as the source of all abundance.

Robert Farrar Capon aptly reminds us, "One real thing is closer to God than all the diagrams in the world."[307] In this sense, *real* food becomes a tangible witness to God's love, logic, and unnecessary goodness, inspiring delight and, in turn, thanksgiving for creation and the Creator who cares for it even in its fallen state. Yet this reflection should also prompt self-examination: do our meals align with this logic? Do they demonstrate a position of participatory membership in this creation, one that promotes thriving families and communities, stewards creation, and supports robust health?

The last part—health—is also a deeply theological concept, though often overlooked as such. What does it mean? What is it for? These are questions for which the secular health field has unsatisfying and superficial answers.

Karl Barth, however, offers a richer perspective by defining health as strength for life. Seen this way, health is infused with purpose, existing not as an end in itself but as a limited good that serves greater Christian virtues. Our unique potential for health is a gift from God, but one that we have both a responsibility and a mandate to promote through our lifestyles. In short, recognizing that our bodies are not our own, but rather God's purchased possession, frames healthy habits as acts of obedience to God's call for stewardship.

Health, seen in this way, can even serve as a form of evangelism. What if, instead of simply presenting a cross-section of a sick world, the body of Christ was marked by robust health? What if the Church, instead of constantly focusing on its own array of diseases, was a physical representation to the rest of the world of the total abundance that Christ offers?

---

307 Capon, *The Supper of the Lamb.*

A candid look at society's failing health reveals a sobering truth: most chronic ailments are both preventable and reversible. Yet this is not the message promoted by our mainstream health establishment. Modern medicine often addresses symptoms in isolation, offering pills or surgeries while sidelining the roles of diet and other lifestyle factors. We are led to believe that our ailments are due to bad genes, unrelated to our choices, or worse, that we can eat whatever we want if we watch the calories (especially saturated fat) and do more cardio. The surprising— and ultimately liberating—truth is that conditions like depression, infertility, fatigue, high blood pressure, excess belly fat, and nine of the ten leading causes of death are often manifestations of the same disease, one over which we have a surprising amount of control.

This disease is metabolic dysfunction, a condition that affects about 88 percent of Americans to some degree.[308] In essence, this overarching condition reflects the body's impaired ability to efficiently convert food into the cellular energy and building blocks that fuel and sustain life. Just as a stem cell can transform into any one of 200 specialized cells, metabolic dysfunction manifests in various ailments, all stemming from the same underlying issues.

At the heart of metabolic dysfunction lies insulin resistance (IR), a critical warning sign and a central driver of numerous health issues. Insulin, a vital metabolic hormone, plays a key role in regulating blood sugar by signaling cells to absorb glucose from the bloodstream to use as energy or store for later use. In a healthy system, this process maintains balanced blood sugar levels and supports cellular function. However, when our cells begin to resist insulin's signal—becoming "deaf" to its instructions—it's a clearly diagnosable marker of metabolic trouble.

Underlying this phenomenon, the two key drivers of metabolic dysfunction—chronic inflammation and oxidative stress—affect nearly every pathway that triggers or exacerbates disease. While these factors can arise from many sources, three contributors stand out: mitochondrial

---

308 Mark J. Lima, Meghan K. Azad, Andrew T. Carey, Kunal K. Ghosh, and Rajesh K. Gupta, "Prevalence of Optimal Metabolic Health in American Adults: National Health and Nutrition Examination Survey 2009–2016," *Metabolism*, vol. 11, no. 1, 2021, pp. 12–20.

dysfunction, leaky gut, and mineral imbalances. By making intentional dietary choices that address these issues, we can significantly optimize metabolic health, stewarding our bodies in a way that reflects God's design for human flourishing.

The first step in this process is simply to reduce or eliminate the things that God didn't design—the food-like substances and additives unfamiliar to our cells. These include, but are not limited to, excessive refined sugars and grains, ultra-processed oils, toxic pesticides and herbicides, and counterproductive vitamin and mineral supplements.

We should strive to replace these modern staples with the foods God designed our bodies to thrive on. This means focusing on high-quality protein to promote muscle health and satiety and ensure our bodies can produce the enzymes, hormones, and neurotransmitters we need. Additionally, we shouldn't shy away from natural, minimally processed fats. Not only do these often accompany protein in nature, but many fatty foods are nutrient dense and abundant in clean-burning energy for our mitochondria. Incorporating fiber and fermented foods supports gut health, while targeting foods or supplements rich in critical micronutrients such as vitamin C complex, magnesium, electrolytes, retinol, B vitamins, and commonly deficient minerals can help optimize every aspect of our metabolic health.

This approach doesn't fit into any trendy box—it's not necessarily ketogenic, vegan, or Mediterranean, and it's far from the seemingly balanced "everything in moderation" philosophy championed by large food corporations. It even diverges from many popular "Christian" diets, such as the "Garden of Eden" and "Maker's" diets, both of which, while certainly well-intentioned and not without their merits, tend to unnecessarily conflate *descriptions* of historical biblical diets with *prescriptions* for modern living.

Although it recognizes the value of eating some foods in their whole forms as provided by God, this plan isn't exactly "Paleo" either. This popular diet strategy helps many people, particularly those with food sensitivities resulting from conventional ultra-processed diets. But we should also be reminded that the Bible frequently references the faithful use of grains like wheat and barley, legumes like beans and lentils, and dairy products like milk and curd, with no mention of food allergies or sensitivities. Bread, for example, though often maligned by modern nutritional advice, can be one of the most nourishing—and tastiest—foods when made whole and fresh, in keeping with God's good design. While today's industrialized food systems may have complicated our relationship with these traditional foods, it would be misguided to suggest that they are inherently harmful.

In short, this diet doesn't err on the side of replacing God's design with humanity's unbridled ingenuity, but it also steers clear of an overly simplistic, hunter-gatherer mindset. Instead, it embraces the principle of stewardship, inviting humanity to glorify God by participating in *His* designs through the agricultural and culinary arts. After all, it's by creating wholesome and enjoyable flavors and dining experiences that we most reflect our own Creator's image.

This principle is beautifully represented in the foods Jesus chose as signs of His body and blood. Neither bread nor wine are "whole foods" per se; both rely on God's raw provision but are transformed through natural processes guided by human skill and effort. This collaboration invites us to recall the sufficiency of God's grace while also exemplifying humanity's active participation in His redemptive work. In this way, these elements serve as a profound reminder that God's partnership with humanity is both a gift and a calling, inviting us to engage with His creation in ways that reflect His logic, love, and abundance.

Understanding *how* and *what* to eat gets us most of the way there, but we can begin to refine our understanding of nutrition by considering *when* to eat. Just as God paired His perfect work with perfect rest in the beginning, a theme of rhythm permeates all of Scripture. Applied to food, this rhythm is modeled in the practice of feasting and fasting, most vividly demonstrated by Jesus Himself. Sometimes the life of the party—frequenting banquets, feeding five thousand, and turning water into wine—our Savior was just as likely to deny food, once fasting in solitude for forty days.

In recent years, various fasting protocols have gained popularity, with growing recognition that the metabolism benefits from occasional rest amid our unprecedented food abundance. But while some modern fasters divorce the practice from its spiritual roots and seek only physical benefits, some Christians take a purely spiritual approach, denying that fasting should also enrich the body. By threading the needle between these extremes, we uncover a holistic practice refined by the saints, validated by modern science, and beneficial to the whole person—mind, body, and spirit—through adherence to daily, weekly, and even seasonal food rhythms.

Incorporating these rhythms into daily life, however, presents its own challenges. Successfully exercising these natural eating rhythms without succumbing to "hanger" and raiding a family-sized bag of Doritos requires metabolic flexibility—the ability to switch seamlessly between glucose burning and fat burning. Cultivating this flexibility depends on consistently providing the right inputs to our cells, which is why adopting a diet built around the five Pillars of the Plate is so important. By focusing on quality protein, natural fats, fiber, fermented foods, and critical vitamins and minerals, we give our bodies the nutrient-dense, satiating foundation needed to balance hormones and promote metabolic resilience.

While these pillars don't inherently favor plant-based or omnivorous approaches, they are more easily incorporated when the latter is the norm. Foods like raw dairy products, eggs, and pasture-raised meats rank among the most nutrient-dense and satiating options available and have been staples in most human cultures throughout history for this very reason.

Still, some Christians reasonably question the place of animal products, especially meat, in the diet. Starting out as eaters of fruit and nuts, then bread, then meat, then only "clean" meat, humanity's relationship with animal foods has certainly evolved over the years. But while all of these shifts reveal something noteworthy (and perhaps debatable) about our anthropology and about the character of God, it's clear that dietary distinctions are no longer relevant under the New Covenant.

While some modern skeptics advocate for animal rights agendas and envision non-violent utopias, a practical understanding of food systems reveals that such ideals are unattainable. Death is an inescapable part of food production—not as a flaw in God's design, but as a sobering reminder of our fallen world. It serves as an object lesson in the spiritual reality that only in death is there hope for new life. Yet, this is not a call for carelessness or complacency in our use of animals for food, nor for treating them as mere commodities subject to cruel confinement or exploitation. On the contrary, faithful Christians are called to honor animals as part of God's creation, allowing them to express their unique glory during their lives as a reflection of the unsurpassable glory of their Creator. Their use for sustenance should be approached only with a spirit of humility and gratitude before the Lord.

In fact, to do so is to round out this paradigm for nutrition. Animals, like it or not, are an integral part of God's logic for food production, which promotes ecosystems rather than monocultures. In the words of Robb Wolf, "Food production is a biological process, and we've turned it into a mechanical one." As we've replaced humans and animals with machines and traded sunlight and soil for petrochemical fertilizers, our modern agricultural system's harmful effects on our health have been matched only by its devastating effects on the environment. By regenerating our land, water, and local ecosystems through the creative application of agricultural systems that utilize both plants and animals, we can meet our nutritional needs while more closely reflecting God's will for His creation.

Adherence to this paradigm is indeed the narrow way compared to the convenience of worldly alternatives. It's a call to live out our faith in *all* of our daily habits—not just in Bible studies or worship services. However, this commitment is not a *substitute* for faith. Our righteousness comes through Christ, not through perfect adherence to dietary protocols. Therefore, our bodies, our food, and our health, though all important, must never become false idols that distract from the other important aspects of a fully human, God-honoring life.

Nor should dietary practices cause division among believers. Paul addresses this directly in Romans 14:1–3:

"As for the one who is weak in faith, welcome him, but not to quarrel over opinions. One person believes he may eat anything, while the weak person eats only vegetables. Let not the one who eats despise the one who abstains, and let not the one who abstains pass judgment on the one who eats, for God has welcomed him."

Paul's guidance is clear: dietary differences should not lead to division or judgment, as God's acceptance is not contingent on food choices.

That said, gentle rebukes may be necessary for believers whose diets are clearly astray. As with any moral aspect of life, there is no kindness in allowing another member of the body to stumble. However, our pursuit of a God-honoring diet must always be tempered with humility and grace, avoiding attitudes of superiority or coercion. We must resist the temptation to become pig-headed or dogmatic about food, for this can lead to unnecessary conflict and distraction from the greater mission of the gospel.

The occasional deep-fried doughnut or drive-through meal doesn't require repentance in sackcloth and ashes. After all, we are embedded within a badly broken food culture, and we should give ourselves and others a little grace in navigating it. But, hopefully, with a healthy dose of knowledge and intentionality, we can rethink our participation in this culture's backwardness.

In doing so, we may find that the act of feeding ourselves doesn't subdue our appetites; it inspires better ones. By delightfully partaking in God's creation and embracing the divine logic intricately woven into it, we cultivate a longing for the eternal banquet that awaits us. And living vibrantly in this hope, we become a testament to the richness of God's design, inspiring others to seek and share in this fuller, more abundant reality for themselves.

Appendix (A Practical Guide)

For some readers, adopting a diet aligned with the principles in this book may require only minor adjustments. For others, it may entail a significant transformation of habits, priorities, and perspectives. Regardless of where you start, the journey toward stewarding your health through a God-honoring approach to nutrition begins with a choice—a commitment to honor God's design for nourishment and human flourishing. But as important as this initial decision is, it's merely the first step. The next step is to develop a clear, actionable plan.

Measure What Matters

In Chapter Four, we emphasized the importance of understanding your current health status. Routine diagnostics are an essential part of this process and can provide valuable insights for tailoring dietary and supplementation strategies to your unique needs. Unfortunately, the standard annual blood panel offered by most physicians is often too limited to give a comprehensive picture of metabolic health. The good news is that holistic practitioners and direct-to-consumer diagnostic services now make comprehensive testing more accessible and affordable than ever.

Routine Blood Work

Aim for semi-annual blood tests that include these key metabolic markers:

Hemoglobin A1c (HbA1c). As discussed in Chapter Seven, this powerhouse marker measures the percentage of glycated red blood cells, offering a three-month snapshot of average blood sugar levels. While values under 5.7 percent are considered normal, aim for no more than 5.4 percent for optimal glucose management.

Fasting Insulin. Rarely tested in conventional settings, fasting insulin can reveal insulin resistance even when fasting glucose appears normal (less than 90 mg/dL). The optimal fasting insulin range is 2–5 µIU/mL, with anything under 10 µIU/mL considered acceptable. For a more complete assessment, use the HOMA-IR formula (discussed in Chapter Seven) to combine fasting glucose and insulin levels.

Triglycerides, HDL, and the Triglycerides/HDL Ratio. These critical biomarkers even appear on the standard lipid panel, but despite their revealing nature, they are rarely discussed by conventional physicians.

- **Triglycerides** measure the amount of "packaged fat" (carried by VLDL particles) circulating in the bloodstream. High levels often indicate excessive carbohydrate intake relative to physical activity. Aim for less than 70 mg/dL; levels above 150 mg/dL almost always indicate insulin resistance.
- Just like HbA1c is like the "area under the curve" for glucose metabolism, **HDL** provides a holistic assessment of lipid metabolism, measuring the body's overall ability to clear excess cholesterol and lipids. Optimal HDL levels range from 50–90 mg/dL.
- **Triglycerides/HDL Ratio** is one of the best proxies for insulin sensitivity and LDL particle size (see Chapter Eight). A ratio below 1.5 signals good insulin sensitivity and predominantly large, buoyant LDL particles (aim for less than one for optimal health). A ratio above two suggests insulin resistance and

a higher presence of small, dense LDL particles, which are linked to cardiovascular risk.

Iron Status. While iron is essential for oxygen transport and energy production, excess iron can contribute to oxidative stress and inflammation. To get a more complete picture of iron status, it's important to monitor not just serum iron, but also ferritin (an iron storage protein), transferrin saturation (the percentage of iron bound to its transport protein), and total iron-binding capacity (TIBC), along with related markers like hemoglobin and hematocrit. Ferritin levels are often considered healthiest in the moderate range, generally below 75–100 ng/mL, though optimal levels may vary by individual and should be interpreted alongside other markers. For those with elevated iron, therapeutic blood donation can be an effective strategy to lower iron stores.

Thyroid Health. Most doctors only test for Thyroid-Stimulating Hormone (TSH) levels and investigate further only if this number is out of range. However, normal TSH levels do not guarantee optimal thyroid function. For a more complete evaluation, include Free T4 (the unbound precursor hormone) and Free T3 (the active hormone), and thyroid antibodies in your panel to assess overall function and screen for autoimmune thyroid disorders like Hashimoto's disease.

High-Sensitivity C-Reactive Protein (hs-CRP). The inflammatory marker, a strong indicator of overall health, should be less than 1.0 mg/L, with lower always being better.

Liver Health Markers. Robert Lustig's mantra for metabolic health is "protect the liver, feed the gut."

- **Aspartate Transaminase (AST) and Alanine Transaminase (ALT)** are proteins that could indicate dysfunctional liver cells, often a result of fatty liver disease and metabolic dysfunction. The optimal range is 0–25 IU/L.
- **Gamma-glutamyl Transferase (GGT)** is an enzyme found throughout the body, but primarily in the liver. Since this

enzyme is used in antioxidant metabolism, its presence is an indirect marker of oxidation. The optimal range is 3–30 U/L.

Hair Tissue Mineral Analysis (HTMA)

HTMA complements bloodwork by providing insights into long-term trends in mineral status. This test is unique in that it measures mineral levels at the cellular level, often a better indicator of chronic deficiencies or toxicities. It's also less invasive and more affordable than blood work, typically needing to be repeated only every 1–2 years. Examples of HTMA insights include:

- The **Calcium/Magnesium ratio** helps to reveal your metabolic efficiency and stress adaptation.
- The **Sodium/Potassium ratio** reflects adrenal and kidney function, cellular hydration, and energy production.
- The **Calcium/Phosphorus ratio** reveals a person's metabolic "type" (slow or fast oxidizer).

Consider consulting a holistic health practitioner trained in the "Root Cause Protocol," who can help analyze these ratios and guide you toward better mineral balance.

Adjust Your Diet and Supplement as Necessary

Armed with a clear snapshot of your unique health condition, you can implement targeted lifestyle changes to address suboptimal metabolic function. Some principles apply broadly, such as managing refined sugars and grains, eliminating ultra processed oils, toxic agricultural chemicals, and unnecessary vitamins and minerals, and building around the five Pillars of the Plate—quality protein, natural fats, fiber, fermented foods, and targeted vitamins and minerals. Aligning meals to promote a healthy circadian rhythm and incorporating occasional weekly or seasonal cleanses can further refine this framework.

Within this foundation, however, there is ample room for personalization. For example, someone with significant metabolic dysfunction might consider severely reducing carbohydrate intake for a while. Some might adopt a two-meal-per-day plan to extend their daily fasting window, while individuals with leptin resistance (diagnosable through blood work) might prioritize an early, high-protein breakfast to signal to the body that it is adequately nourished.

As previously discussed, supplements may be necessary to address nutrient deficiencies and counteract the many assaults of modern life.

Foundational Supplements

Supplement routines should also be intentional and directed toward specific outcomes. While broad-spectrum multivitamins often do more harm than good, several foundational supplements support general metabolic health. These include:

Magnesium. Aim to consume roughly 3–5 mg of elemental magnesium per pound of body weight per day, as discussed in Chapter Eight. When supplementing, choose bioavailable forms like magnesium malate or glycinate. While magnesium threonate has become popular for its ability to cross the blood brain barrier and promote cognitive health, it is less effective at boosting general magnesium levels.

Vitamin C Complex. Also highlighted in Chapter 8, consider adding 300–500 mg of high-quality vitamin C complex to your routine. Choose food-based sources like Acerola Cherry, Amla Berry, and Camu Camu Berry, and avoid synthetic ascorbic acid.

Electrolytes. As noted in Chapter Eight, sodium isn't the villain it's often made out to be. Ensuring adequate sodium intake reduces stress on the kidneys and promotes overall hydration. Include a sugar-free electrolyte mix for daily use and to maintain hydration during exercise. Brands like LMNT, Redmond's Re-Lyte, and many others provide balanced formulas that include potassium and magnesium for comprehensive electrolyte support.

Cod Liver Oil (CLO). High-quality CLO is a rich source of omega-3 fatty acids (DHA and EPA), has high levels of retinol (vitamin A), and comes with some vitamin D in the appropriate ratio for optimal absorption. These vitamins must work together to provide their full range of benefits.

Bee Pollen. Known as nature's multivitamin, bee pollen is a nutrient-dense superfood packed with B vitamins, vitamin C, vitamin E, carotenoids, selenium, and zinc. Its versatility allows it to be added to smoothies, yogurts, or other foods. Look for brands offering third-party tested products.

Other General Supplements to Consider

In addition to the foundational options, these other food-based supplements may be worth considering based on diagnostic insights or other needs:

Protein Powder. Protein powder is an excellent option for anyone struggling to meet their daily protein needs through diet alone, especially those eating fewer than three meals a day, individuals who are physically active, and the elderly. High-quality protein powders are available in both plant- and animal-based forms, but the key is to choose one with wholesome origins and minimal ingredients.

Desiccated Beef Organs. If offal isn't your thing, then consider adding a desiccated organ supplement to your routine. Liver is a well-rounded nutrient powerhouse, offering retinol, several B vitamins, copper, heme iron, choline, and selenium. Desiccated heart tends to benefit cardiovascular and cellular health, with high concentrations of coenzyme Q10 (CoQ10), B vitamins, zinc, taurine, heme iron, and phosphorus. Not to be overlooked, kidney is particularly beneficial for detoxification and immune support, providing vitamin B_{12}, selenium, zinc, and glutathione. Look for delicately processed, pasture-raised sources with no fillers or additives.

Collagen. Collagen is the most abundant protein in the body, playing a vital role in maintaining joint health, skin elasticity, and the strength of the gut lining. It provides structural support for connective tissues, promotes healthy cartilage, and may aid in gut healing by supporting the integrity of the intestinal barrier. Collagen is naturally found in bone broth, animal connective tissues, and minimally processed collagen powders, yet it is often lacking in modern diets due to the decline of traditional cooking practices like slow-simmered broths and nose-to-tail eating.

Basil Seeds. Basil seeds are similar to chia seeds in that they absorb liquid and expand with a gel-like substance that forms around them. But while chia seeds have some anti-nutrient compounds that may cause irritation, basil seeds lack these compounds and pack even more of a nutrient punch. Two tablespoons provide 15 grams of prebiotic fiber, omega-3 fatty acids (ALA), and several minerals. Hydrated basil seeds work well in overnight oats, puddings, or beverages.

A functional health practitioner can help you interpret your test results and determine whether more targeted supplements may be appropriate—such as iodine for thyroid support, selenium for antioxidant protection, or methylated B vitamins (especially for those with the MTHFR gene variant, which may impair folate metabolism and methylation pathways). In some cases, practitioners may also recommend therapeutic peptides (such as BPC-157 for tissue repair or thymosin alpha-1 for immune modulation) or nutraceuticals like berberine and N-acetyl cysteine (NAC) to further enhance metabolic function and resilience.

By understanding your unique health profile through targeted diagnostics, adjusting your diet to focus on nutrient dense foods, and filling any gaps with carefully chosen supplements, you can take meaningful steps toward optimizing your metabolic health. Remember, this journey is not about perfection but faithful progress, empowered by the wisdom of God's design.

Go Deeper, Reach Further!

Thank you for reading *Nourished by Design*. If you've found encouragement, clarity, or conviction in these pages, there's more waiting for you.

Download Your Free Devotional Guide + Tools

At **NourishedByDesignBook.com**, you'll find a free, printable 5-Step Devotional Companion Guide, designed to expand upon this appendix and help you implement the book's key principles. You'll also get access to bonus tools and resources to support your ongoing health journey.

Leave a Review, Change a Life

Each new review for this book could help it reach hundreds of additional people—people like you, looking for a deeper faith and a healthier life aligned with God's design.

If this book has blessed or challenged you in any way, here's how you can help:

1. Go to **NourishedByDesignBook.com**
2. Click "Purchase or Leave a Review on Amazon"
3. Click "Write a Review" and share a few honest thoughts

Your simple act of leaving a review will make a massive difference in the lives of others. It gives them confidence to take a chance on this book—and opens the door to real transformation.

Thank you for taking this small step to help others experience the blessing of being nourished by God's design.

– Andy Felton

Acknowledgements

I am neither a theologian nor a medical doctor, and in many ways this proved to be an advantage. It allowed me to approach the issues in this book with an open mind and a sensitivity to varying levels of understanding. But it has also left me deeply dependent on the work of others—authors, researchers, and thinkers—whose ideas and insights have provided me with guidance and inspiration. Without their contributions, this book would not have been possible.

First and foremost, I owe a great debt to Leon Kass, whose classic work, *The Hungry Soul*, offered a profound anthropological perspective on the human person and our relationship with food. His analysis of the Jewish dietary laws, the supremacy of form in the human body, and the significance of upright posture—drawing on the legacy of Erwin Straus—shaped much of my thinking.

Joel Salatin, a pioneer in regenerative agriculture, also had a significant influence through his book, *The Marvelous Pigness of Pigs*. His idea that the material aspects of God's creation serve as object lessons in spiritual realities was both convicting and enlightening. I am especially grateful for Joel's generosity in reading my early manuscript and writing a thoughtful foreword in his characteristically colorful style.

On the theology of the body, I drew heavily on the work of John Paul II, complemented by John Kleinig's Protestant perspective on the topic. Norman Wirzba's *Food and Faith* introduced me to the concept of Eucharistic eating and provided an insightful Christian framework for understanding food. Jay Richards's *Eat, Fast, Feast* was another invaluable resource, combining modern scientific research with Christian tradition to illuminate the practice of fasting. Finally, Robert Farrar Capon's lighthearted yet profound culinary reflection, *The Supper of the Lamb*, complimented many of these themes and provided an almost endless supply of insightful quotes. These authors provided the intellectual foundation for much of this book.

I am also grateful to several friends, family members, and mentors who offered their support and insight along the way. Jeff Pearson provided thoughtful feedback on several chapters, recommended excellent resources, and shared his deep knowledge of Roman Catholic doctrine, especially as it relates to the Lord's Supper. Parker Landis, a pastor at Crossroads Bible Church, also gave generously of his time to critique my early drafts and offer invaluable encouragement.

Finally, I want to thank my beautiful wife, Lindsey, for her unwavering support and honest feedback throughout this project. Writing a book while raising two toddlers was no small feat, and her patience, love, and partnership made all the difference.

I am deeply grateful to all of these individuals and many others not named. Their contributions have enriched this book in ways I could not have accomplished alone.